Aroma, Aromatherapy and Trauma

T0385381

by the same author

Working with Unusual Essential Oils
Helen Nagle-Smith
Foreword by Jennifer Peace Rhind
ISBN 978 1 80501 179 8
eISBN 978 1 80501 180 4

of related interest

Essential Oils (Fully Revised and Updated 3rd Edition)
A Comprehensive Handbook for Aromatic Therapy (3rd Edition)
Jennifer Peace Rhind
ISBN 978 1 78775 229 0
eISBN 978 0 85701 343 9

The Personalised Consultation in Aromatherapy
A Practitioner Guide
Annie Prince
ISBN 978 1 80501 146 0
eISBN 978 1 80501 147 7

Integrating Clinical Aromatherapy in Palliative Care
Carol Rose
Foreword by Rhiannon Lewis
ISBN 978 1 83997 160 0
eISBN 978 1 83997 161 7

Contemporary French Aromatherapy
A Pharmacological and Therapeutic Guide to 100 Essential Oils
Dominique Baudoux
Foreword by Kurt Schnaubelt
ISBN 978 1 78775 026 5
eISBN 978 1 78775 027 2

Aroma, Aromatherapy and Trauma

Helen Nagle-Smith

Foreword by Rhiannon Lewis

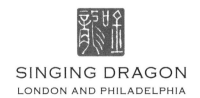

SINGING DRAGON

LONDON AND PHILADELPHIA

First published in Great Britain in 2025 by Singing Dragon,
an imprint of Jessica Kingsley Publishers
Part of John Murray Press

1

Disclaimer: The information, formulas and ideas in this book are not intended as a
substitute for medical advice or care. Any application of the ideas, information and
formulas in this book are done at the sole risk of the reader. It is up to the reader
to individually assess any contraindications with any essential oil, carrier oil, CO_2
extract, hydrolat or other aromatic ingredient mentioned. If you are not a qualified
aromatherapist, you should seek advice from a qualified aromatherapist before using
essential oils. The author does not promote ingestion or internal use of essential oils.

A CIP catalogue record for this title is available from the
British Library and the Library of Congress

ISBN 978 1 80501 279 5
eISBN 978 1 80501 280 1

Printed and bound by CPI Group (UK) Ltd, Croydon, CR0 4YY

Jessica Kingsley Publishers' policy is to use papers that are natural,
renewable and recyclable products and made from wood grown in
sustainable forests. The logging and manufacturing processes are expected
to conform to the environmental regulations of the country of origin.

Singing Dragon
Carmelite House
50 Victoria Embankment
London EC4Y 0DZ

www.singingdragon.com

John Murray Press
Part of Hodder & Stoughton Limited
An Hachette UK Company

The authorised representative in the EEA is Hachette Ireland,
8 Castlecourt Centre, Dublin 15, D15 XTP3, Ireland (email: info@hbgi.ie)

To those who have shared their experiences with me along the decades and from whom I have learned so much, and to those who have worked so tirelessly to demonstrate the impact of trauma on humanity and how we can do things differently.

Contents

Foreword

Since the late 1990s, a clear framework for trauma-informed care has emerged and spread across healthcare, education, criminal justice and social services worldwide. The trauma-informed approach recognizes and responds to the impact of trauma on individuals, emphasizing safety, empowerment and healing. What is more, trauma-informed care addresses the social, cultural and historical contexts of trauma, helping to reduce stigma and bias. More recently, this framework has gradually extended and become integrated into the world of complementary and alternative therapy provision.

Whenever a person reaches out for therapy, care or assistance – be that mainstream or complementary – cultivating a safe therapeutic environment is key for improved outcomes. The trauma-informed therapist employs special skills, attention and sensitivity and enhances the impact of the care provided. They ensure that the therapeutic encounter is both physically and emotionally safe and prevent any practices that might unintentionally trigger trauma reactions or escalate distress.

Feeling safe in therapy also necessitates choice, control and the need to be truly heard by the practitioner. Feeling safe fosters resilience, enabling people to regain control and take positive steps toward healing. Cultivating a safe therapeutic encounter is thus key for all interactions.

In the case of aromatherapy provision, depending on individual circumstances and experiences, a particular aroma may be perceived either as a trigger to a negative or traumatic response or as a bridge to a safe, familiar and soothing experience. The line between these two perceptions and responses is fine and fragile. Aromas always lead to instant like/dislike responses. Thus, there is great responsibility on the part of the aromatherapist to ensure that negative triggering is avoided and that positive responses are always the desired outcome.

It is often the case that in the safety and sanctity of the therapeutic encounter, the individual accesses the opportunity to voice, express and process traumatic experiences. It is essential that the therapist is equipped with core skills to safely accompany and support the person, should this arise, and to recognize when referral or other support is required.

Being trauma-informed also helps the therapist to avoid burnout through helping them be better equipped to manage the challenges of working with trauma survivors. Reflective practices, mentoring and clinical supervision are currently rare in the aromatherapy world – an issue that is clearly highlighted in this book.

Until now, no text or written guidance on trauma-informed care has existed for aromatherapists or aromatherapy educators. This timely landmark text therefore fills an important need for the evolution and continued integration of this gentle healing art and science within health and social care.

The author has acquired many years of experience in this field, having worked with individuals and families affected by emotional, mental and physical trauma and witnessed their far-reaching impact on health and behaviour. She has delved deeply into the research and practices concerning trauma-informed care and has successfully and calmly woven these into her own practice as a professional aromatherapist.

Through this remarkable text that explores difficult topics with great clarity using a conversational and engaging style, she now provides insight, perspective, research and guidance to other practitioners, encouraging them to work safely and effectively and with greater awareness regarding historical and recent trauma experiences. Drawing on her own work as well as that of other professional aromatherapists around the world, she illustrates the text with aromatherapy-specific cases and thinking points and offers an extremely pragmatic exploration of a complex and sensitive area of therapy.

This book is essential reading for anyone in the aromatherapy world, from the student aromatherapist at the start of their aromatic career to the seasoned practitioner for whom perhaps the framework for trauma-informed care did not exist at the time of their own training. I am honoured to write this foreword.

Rhiannon Lewis

Acknowledgements

I have learned a lot about trauma from many people in my lifetime, especially my clients (in both my careers), and I am thankful for all they have taught me. It was (and is) an honour to be part of their journey.

As you will see throughout the book, many aromatherapists have been kind enough to share their experiences with me and allowed me to include them in the book. Caren Benstead, Cathy Skipper, Cynthia Tamlyn, Denise Cusack, Donna Robbins, Elaine Le Feuvre, Elizabeth Ashley, Elizabeth Guthrie, Florian Birkmayer, Fusako Takada, Jane Lawson, Jonathan Benavides, Lora Cantele, Madeleine Kerkhof, Natascha Köhler, Nicole Boukhalil, Rehne Burge, Saboohi Kahn, Sue Adlam, Sue Jenkins and Victoria Plum, thank you for sharing your experiences and wisdom, and thank you for all the aromatic work you do.

My journey as a student aromatherapist started in 2005 when I was a student at the Institute for Traditional and Herbal Medicine (ITHMA). The experience entrenched my love of aromatherapy, and I realized I had found my vocation and come home.

I am very grateful for the support and wisdom of many aromatherapy friends around the world, in particular Caren Benstead, Deby Atterby, Elaine Le Feuvre, Elizabeth Ashley, Lora Cantele, Madeleine Kerkhof, Rhiannon Lewis and Trish Drane, thank you for always encouraging me. Thank you to Ian Cambray-Smith and Elizabeth Ashley for 'test reading' certain chapters as I was finishing the book. I especially need to recognize Jennifer Peace Rhind, who has been such a supportive writing buddy and mentor even though we have never met. She has helped me pick myself up and carry on when I have been struggling to write, listened to my ideas and helped me explore themes on numerous occasions.

Thank you to all the team at Singing Dragon, in particular my Editor Carole McMurray who recognized the importance of the subject and always has such faith in me to transform the proposal into a book.

Finally, thanks to Paul and Kate. You understand when I dive down the rabbit hole of writing, and support my endeavours however laborious they are. None of this would happen without you.

About the author

After a previous career in the voluntary sector, delivering, shaping and managing information and counselling services, Helen Nagle-Smith (BA, MIFPA) trained with the Institute for Traditional and Herbal Medicine (ITHMA) in London and qualified in 2006. She runs her own aromatherapy and massage practice, is an aromatherapy educator and writer, and talks internationally.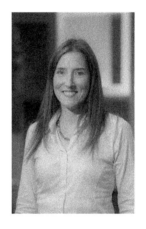

In 2020, Helen wrote *Working with Unusual Oils: An aromatic journey with lesser-known essential oils – Volume 1*, covering 18 more unusual oils. In 2024, her second book, *Working with Unusual Essential Oils* (published by Singing Dragon), covered 40 lesser-known essential oils. Helen has written numerous articles (including peer-reviewed ones) for several international aromatherapy journals, including the *International Journal of Professional Holistic Aromatherapy*, *Aromatika*, *In Essence* and *Aromatherapy Today*.

She lives in Buckinghamshire, UK with her husband and daughter. When not working, Helen can be found with her family, walking her dog, working at her allotment, reading, occasionally baking, and catching up with friends.

To get in touch or find out more about Helen's latest projects go to www. aromatherapywithhelen.com or email info@aromatherapywithhelen.com. Helen is currently working on her next book.

If you have enjoyed this book, please leave a review.

Introduction

> **Gentle reminder/content warning**
> Go gently as you read this book, and if it taps into anything for you, or becomes too much, know that you can put the book to one side. Do what you need to do to look after yourself and feel safe. You can return to it later if you wish to.

Trauma has been referred to as a 'defining health threat' of the 21st century (Porges & Porges, 2023) and quite rightly so. By not exploring it, we allow those who experience trauma to continue to feel shame, guilt and embarrassment. Its consequences not only affect the individual but also ripple through society. Useful definitions are hard to find, but generally anything horrific that completely overwhelms us in a way that makes it hard to manage day-to-day life may be considered traumatic.

Trauma can turn worlds upside down and inside out. It changes the way people view the world and feel about themselves and others (van der Kolk, 2014). It can result in many symptoms, including experiencing intrusive thoughts and memories, nightmares, flashbacks, dissociation (so people don't feel as if they are in their bodies, or feel spacey or numb), sleep and memory problems, overwhelming negative feelings, hyperactivity, hypervigilance (feeling 'on edge' or being easily startled), feeling unsafe, emotional or angry outbursts, avoidance of places, people or things, other physical issues such as tinnitus, poor breathing patterns, racing heart, feeling pain and more (PTSDUK, 2023a).

Trauma can change our physiology, making us more prone to illness and disease (Lewis-O'Connor *et al.*, 2019; Katrinli *et al.*, 2022; Maté, 2019; van der Kolk, 2014; Levine, 2018), and can cause changes both in the adult brain (van der Kolk, 2014; Teicher & Samson, 2016; PTSDUK, 2023b) and the child's developing brain (Jeong *et al.*, 2021).

The ripples of trauma flow through society, with many of our societal structures, systems and organizations perpetuating more trauma (Menakem, 2021). Our reactions on a bodily level are often unconscious, and although some of our physiology and behaviours may be shaped by trauma, it does not always feel possible to acknowledge or understand this, for many of us still live in a society where it is hard to talk about pain. Having a 'stiff upper lip' is very British behaviour. It refers to trying not to cry and carrying on as though nothing has happened emotionally. Culturally, we are not good at allowing ourselves to feel anguish and despair (I suspect this has ancestral roots in our history of colonialism, slavery and religious persecution, and more latterly the Second World War).

Definitions for trauma are challenging, and the *Diagnostic and Statistical Manual of Mental Disorders* (*DSM-5*) criteria used in many countries can be critiqued. They do not even include complex post-traumatic stress disorder (C-PTSD).

Trauma definitions are often too narrow and pay no attention to systematic trauma that people may experience due to discrimination, such as homophobia, racism or sexism. These definitions not only ignore the impact of society and culture, but also trauma which may happen in utero, and in the first few years of a child's life (I will unpick this more in Chapter 3).

I thought I knew a lot about trauma from my first career and other experiences, but writing this book has taught me that I had more to learn. I knew the parts I witnessed, heard and sometimes felt – the bits of life I wanted to leave me alone but which I couldn't always ignore, memories I put in a box, high on a shelf in the warehouse of my mind. For a long time, like many, I saw trauma as something that played out psychologically. Psychological support and help from family and friends seemed to be the answer. I certainly didn't appreciate its link to long-term health conditions, and the multiple ways in which the body stored trauma until I became an aromatherapist and learned to massage, nor did I know that it changes our brain and can even alter how (and if) we smell.

Even though I have a sociology degree, as I grew older, I spent less and less time considering the role of society, neglecting perhaps to understand how we facilitate trauma within it and the systems we use. By not truly addressing, exploring and acknowledging this existence we allow its impact to continue, and we make it hard for people to be supported in moving towards a place of post-traumatic growth. As a society, we have a long way to go. I hope that this book adds to the conversation, and that it makes you want to explore further.

In 2020, while writing my first aromatherapy book, I was struck by how many of the essential oils I was writing about were indicated for trauma. I was writing during a UK lockdown, created by a global pandemic, so this was hardly surprising. We were experiencing collective trauma across the world. As I pondered this thought, I carried on writing, teaching online, making up aromatherapy products and offering online self-massage and relaxation sessions for clients. While I was offering my clients the power of aroma and somatics as a way of coping, helping them with what was happening in the world, unwittingly, I was also supporting myself through this.

Before becoming an aromatherapist, I'd worked in the voluntary sector in a variety of paid roles and had also been a volunteer for a listening service. My time was spent in information and counselling services, and, over the years, I worked with countless young people, young adults and families who experienced numerous different forms of trauma. In my first job, I worked with many adolescents and young women into their twenties, who had experienced sexual violence, domestic violence, abuse within the home (physical, emotional and sexual) or bullying. Later, I would see people's lives shaped by other traumas such as medical procedures, illness and life-changing accidents.

Trauma can inform how we respond to the signals our senses pick up. Sounds, sights, tactile sensations, touch, even tastes may be unconsciously triggering. Over the years, several people mentioned to me that the smell of something could be a trigger. It could bring on fast, involuntary and powerful reactions such as flashbacks, a freeze response, dizziness or a wave of nausea. This was truly terrifying for people and at this point I began to comprehend that aroma and trauma were heavily entwined; however, I didn't really work with smell until I changed careers.

When I became an aromatherapist I wanted to approach my work in a person-centred way, using essential oils holistically to help people with where they were at emotionally, physically and spiritually. Over the years, trauma has continued to enter my workplace, not in a huge way, but often unexpectedly. Sometimes when I meet a client for the first time they may disclose a past trauma, perhaps they are awaiting a PTSD diagnosis or referral. In most instances, this isn't the case and they tend to divulge information over a period of months and years as they get to know me and I become a safe confidant.

I have also realized that many people don't attribute the word *trauma* to their experience. I have found this is especially true of older clients in their sixties, seventies and eighties, who grew up with emotional neglect and abuse. Instead, they may use words like 'difficult childhood', 'hard time growing up', or say that a parent was cruel, belittling or never kind.

It is not up to me or anyone else to tell someone how they should define their experiences, but it is important to acknowledge and understand that different words may be used but the outcomes (especially on someone's health) may be similar. Whether a trauma such as childhood abuse or neglect is acknowledged or not, the wound is there all the same.

Like many other professionals, as aromatherapists we know we can't separate the mind from the body or vice versa, and most of us don't aim to. We wish to work holistically. We see mind, body and soul as intrinsically linked, and anecdotally often see links between a medical condition starting and things that happen in a person's life. Recently, a client told me about a particular experience which she described as traumatic. I listened and said that her experience sounded as if it had been extremely hard for her. She nodded and then told me that a complementary health professional had recently told her she had noticed a pattern of multiple traumas across her life; she had sensitively asked my client if she thought there may be some connection. By asking this question, the conversation had been started. The external acknowledgement and validation gave my client permission to explore this.

It is important to understand that because a trauma has occurred this does not automatically mean a person will become ill or develop a long-term medical condition. There are lots of variables at large here. It also does not mean that a long-term medical condition is psychosomatic or imagined. To suggest this is failing to understand the biological implications of trauma on the human body, and it is potentially diminishing.

Many of my fellow aromatherapists state that they are seeing more people experiencing secondary trauma (sometimes called indirect or vicarious trauma). This normally refers to people who are experiencing trauma because of working with people who are traumatized. The name has its limitations (as we will see later), but also helps us to understand that trauma is much more pervasive than originally thought. COVID-19 has impacted mental health, with research showing higher proportions of the population vulnerable to PTSD since the pandemic, with medical, health and social workers being particularly impacted (Herz, 2021; Langley-Brady *et al.*, 2023).

Conversations around trauma today are increasingly focused on polyvagal theory and the usefulness of breath work and somatic exercises (Langley-Brady *et al.*, 2023). These are fascinating to me because I am a body worker, and much of it relates to what I see play out for people in both this career and my previous one. Certainly, such work can inform those of us working with clients. Yet as an aromatherapist, I remain deeply frustrated that our sense of smell is still so often neglected.

Our sense of smell seems to walk in the shadow of vision and hearing. In one study, Herz and Bajec (2022) found that the sense of smell was seen as massively less important than sight and hearing and one quarter of college students said they would give up their sense of smell over and above keeping their phone. This says a lot about the power (and addictive quality) of technology, but also the lack of importance that smell seems to hold for many.

As an aromatherapist, I deeply appreciate how aroma can be a positive anchor. Due to the close link between our olfactory system and the limbic area in the brain, aromas can remind us of happy memories or times we felt safe. Essential oils can also help us practically with aspects such as memory recall and relaxation (Rhind, 2020) and they can be a support to our nervous system (Langley-Brady *et al.*, 2023). There is more to aromatherapy than a pleasing scent (Conrad, 2019).

While there is an increasing body of research demonstrating the positive impact of essential oils on our mind and our body (Rhind, 2020), there is little pertaining to essential oils or aromatherapy and trauma.

There is some research around post-traumatic stress disorder (normally called PTSD or PTS), and I will refer to some of this throughout the book. However, I try to balance research and statistics with experiences of other people working with trauma and aroma, or my own client work and experiences. These give more detail, and while many of the people mentioned did not have a formal PTSD diagnosis, this does not mean they had not experienced, or were not experiencing, trauma.

Research and trauma statistics normally rely on data of those who have a diagnosis of PTSD, because of the need to be able to measure and reproduce this. The pitfall of this is that we underestimate the true extent of trauma for individuals and larger society.

In the field of aromatherapy, larger, more robust studies and more longitudinal research are required. In our treatment rooms, aromatherapists typically blend between three and five essential oils. I most commonly work with three at any given time. This allows a synergy, and we know that adding oils together sometimes enhances their effects (Rhind, 2016). Much of the research regarding how they impact our mental and physical health is done on single essential oils. Understandably, this reduces variables, but it would be interesting to see if we can bridge this gap.

For me, researching the process of olfaction (smell) and unravelling the role and relationship smell and trauma can have with each other has been fascinating, and exploring how we smell and the social, historical, political and cultural context of this has been utterly absorbing.

As I broke the book down into sections, I became intrigued to think about how we deliver our aromatherapy services. Cycling back in my mind to my previous career where I was responsible for shaping client services, I realized I had more work to do in becoming more trauma informed, and shaping my own practice. I started to research what was happening in health and social care services. What aspects of developing trauma-informed services could we bring from this world into our model of working as aromatherapists? What did we have in our tool kits that could be most useful and how could we best support our clients and ourselves?

Many of us have worked hard to build up aromatherapy businesses and careers. Being self-employed (as the majority of aromatherapists are) is not for the faint hearted. It requires passion, dedication, tenacity and long hours. In tackling this subject, it made me question so many of the fundamentals that we have in place. Are our intake/consultation forms adequate? How do we maintain our boundaries? What can we do if a client is impacted or triggered while they are with us? Have we addressed our own trauma histories and how do we react when our clients bring something to the treatment room that is close to our own experience? Do we know when to refer on? During crisis aromatherapy work, are we able to offer the same levels of protection to our clients and ourselves?

It soon became evident that I also needed to explore what work we need to do with ourselves in healing our own wounds. In my previous career, this was understood and acknowledged, but in the aromatherapy field it is rarely discussed. Perhaps in wanting to write this I had wounds that needed work? In all honesty, this unconsciously travelled with me for a while before I dared to acknowledge it. We cannot explore supporting others in their world if we are scared to look at our own, and I firmly believe that we all have trauma across our lifespan and the lives of our families, friends and ancestors, for that is part of being human.

Sharing other aromatherapists' stories of working with clients who were experiencing trauma or who had trauma histories felt crucial. We can learn so much from each other and pave the way for future generations.

I knew writing this book would feel like an enormous mountain to climb. It would be difficult, uncomfortable and messy. I procrastinated for a few years, unwilling to take myself there. Now it is here I feel very differently about it. This book has convinced me that there is so much more we can do to help each other when there is trauma. Aroma and aromatherapy can be wonderful supports.

There is a palpable risk that in writing about trauma you become despondent because it inevitably means touching on some of the worst traits of humanity, but there is always hope and there is always the possibility that we can move forwards, into a new way of being. Sometimes lived experience of trauma drives people into specific careers or directions, enabling them to take part in creating positive change. Post-traumatic growth is something I will touch on later in the book.

Please note that I tend to use the term 'lived experience'. There is a vast terminology if you have experienced trauma. 'Trauma survivors', 'victims', 'warriors' or having 'lived experience' are probably the most heard terms. I do not think it is up to me or anyone else to declare that any one of these is right or wrong, but it is important that people use terminology that sits with their experience.

This book isn't here to be a definitive guide on trauma or aromatherapy or olfaction. Instead, it is a meeting point where these three things intersect. If you have an interest in any of these three subjects, then this book is for you.

Now is the time to meaningfully address the topic of trauma and its relationship with aroma, reclaim the importance of smell and understand how aromatherapy may be of benefit. Let us shine a light on how essential oils and other aromatic allies can bring meaningful support to our lives, especially during the more difficult times.

Finally, I want to honour those who have spoken to me about their own trauma histories, the aromatherapists who work around the globe supporting traumatized clients, and those who have already started paving this path and discussing trauma within our profession. I also wish to acknowledge the contribution of those who research olfaction. All of you are precious and I thank you.

CHAPTER 1

The role of aroma in our lives

Smell is a potent wizard that transports you across thousands of miles and all the years you have lived.

Helen Keller

For most of us, smell is part of our everyday life. It is hidden in the fabric of life, interwoven in our day, often unappreciated and taken for granted. The process of smell (olfaction) relates to so much of our lives, including our biology, physiology, neurology, sociability, psychology, psyche, cognition, well-being, memories and emotions.

Smell is often considered to be the poor relation of the senses, and in modern Western life our visual and auditory senses have dominated and are more favoured (Barwich, 2020). Although there are cultures that give smell a much greater significance than the Western world (Herz & Bajec, 2022), these are few and far between.

It is intriguing to see how little language we have for smell when we compare this to other senses such as sight. Even in aromatherapy we sometimes struggle with words to describe smell and will often fall on those used to describe wines or food. The language we use is complicated because it is sometimes ambiguous, or it covers a wide range of aromas. If I told you I could smell a citrus aroma, I could be describing many things – mango, orange, lemon or a number of other fruits. They all smell wildly different and yet they could all be described as having a citrus scent. Our language for smell could be improved if it became more sophisticated. However, if I asked you to think of something that smelt 'lemony', you would know exactly what I meant. Your home is likely to contain something that has a lemony aroma, whether it is sweets, washing-up liquid, bathroom or floor cleaning products, reed diffusers, perfumes or cosmetics. It is a popular and easily recognized aroma. Some lucky readers would even be able to conjure a memory of that smell in their mind, (until very recently I assumed everyone could do this, but this is not the case).

How we consider smell has changed over time, and in different periods it has been used to vilify. Ward (2023) reminds us it has all too often been associated with disease and illness, derided as being primitive. 'Bad' smells in history been attributed to poverty and the poor, and to jobs no one wanted, such as being a fuller or tanner (both jobs used urine). Cobb (2020) informs us that access to pleasant aromas and perfumes and the ability to keep oneself clean were far more possible when you had money and power.

Even religion has harnessed the sense of smell and there are a surprising number of references to smell in the Bible. For example:

> But thanks be to God who always leads us in triumphant procession in Christ. And through us spreads everywhere the fragrance of the knowledge of him. For we are to God the aroma of Christ among those who are being saved and those who are perishing. To the one we are the smell of death; to the other the fragrance of life. And who is equal to such a task? (2 Corinthians 2:14–16 New International Version: Holy Bible, 2011)

In Ephesians 5:2 (New International Version), Christ is referred to as a 'fragrant' offering. Incense has been used in religious and spiritual ceremonies for hundreds and hundreds of years.

Barwich (2020) tells us that in medieval times, odours acted as 'moral signatures', and sins and senses became linked. It is intriguing to see how rotten aromas have often been associated with the devil, evil, hell and ungodliness. In Dante's *Inferno* we see lurid descriptions of the stench of hell and rotting flesh. Smells tend to be labelled as 'good' or 'bad' and as such those in power can use them to separate themselves from the masses.

Years ago, Greek and Roman philosophers theorized that atoms had particular shapes. Pleasant smells were made from pleasing, round atoms and sharp or bitter aromas came from pointy ones (Cobb, 2020; Totaro & Wainright, 2022). As a synesthete (meaning I experience a convergence of two or more senses), I find this fascinating. Aroma taking a visual element brings a smile to my face, because in my mind essential oils often have a colour or colours attached to their scent. Interestingly, Cobb (2020) notes that these philosophers were on the right track, as it appears there is a link between the molecular configuration of a smell and our perception of it.

While we probably know less about smell than our other senses, research on the subject has gained momentum in more recent decades, especially since Buck and Axel (1991) discovered that olfactory receptor genes existed.

Outside the olfactory scientific community, the world finally woke up to the importance of smell during COVID-19. Many people experienced smell loss (anosmia) for the first time. Aromatherapists and anyone whose profession relied on smell were particularly frightened of losing their sense of smell. For some, lack of or altered smell may be part of long COVID. Anosmia can also develop due to head trauma, illness, smoking, medical treatment, medication, use of illegal drugs or poisoning, and it is thought to affect around 5% of the population (Boesveldt & Parma, 2021).

Most people can tell you relatively quickly of their favourite smells. These are sometimes culturally specific. I have a neighbour who grows a selection of beautiful pink roses from David Austin nurseries. They grow up a fence in his front garden and pop their flowery blooms through the trellis gaps. When passing, I can't help but stop and smell the delicate sweet aroma. It reminds me of summer and warmth. If you recognize and enjoy the aroma of roses, reading this will probably make you smile, give you a warm fuzzy feeling inside, or bring an image or memory to mind. If you were brought up having never smelt a flower or roses it would be meaningless to you.

Herz (2021) reminds us that various cultures have different interpretations of scent, even though some scents are very common in multiple cultures and countries. Rosewater is commonly used in many countries, and it may be used in multiple ways, for example as a perfume or in food (Lewis & Ossola, 2023). Aromatherapist and herbalist Denise Cusack told me how she liked to use Rose (*Rosa damascena*) essential oil for aroma inhalers when she was working with groups of refugees from Afghanistan. Denise noted that in her culture (the USA), the scent of roses may be seen as cloying, old and unpleasant. For Afghan refugee women, she found Rose essential oil to be a strong familial cultural aroma that was comforting and calming. Even using the tiniest amount of it gleaned positive responses.

I was intrigued to find out what the most desirable smells are and stumbled across research by Arshamian *et al.* (2022). They claimed that cultural variance does exist (e.g. fermented fish may be seen as a delicacy in Sweden and is generally liked by Scandinavians but normally disliked by other cultures) but is lower than previously thought. They studied 225 people from nine diverse cultures (including non-Western hunter gatherers in differing environments such as coastal or rainforest regions, or mountain communities) and asked them to rank ten smells in order of most to least pleasant. Surprisingly, they stated that cultural variance only accounted for 6%. They concluded that individual smell preference and physicochemical properties of the molecules was markedly more important than cultural variance. The most preferred smell was 4-Hydroxy-3-methoxybenzaldehyde (Vanillin), which has a creamy vanilla aroma. Ethyl butanoate (commonly known as Ethyl butyrate) came second, with its fruity, juicy aroma.

Arshamian et al. (2022) suggested that personal preference may be due to learning or genetics (though one could argue learning may be influenced by culture). They postulated that the reason some aromas may be favoured over others may be due to evolution and trying to increase human survival. They don't expand too much on this, but it is interesting that the top two aromas are something many people associate as being food-like aromas.

We understand that our noses have always alerted us to beauty (e.g. the smell of a flower), to food (e.g. fruit) and to danger (e.g. the smell of sickness, fire, rotten food and gas). However, there are intriguing variations in our reaction to this which are hard to ignore. Cobb (2020) cited the work of Hoover et al. (2015), who looked at a large sample of over 1000 indigenous people across the world. They posited that olfactory gene variations may account for differing reactions to the smell of androsterone. People who found the aroma sweet seemed to have eaten pork, yet people who had the ancestral African form of the gene seemed to find the aroma distasteful. This implies that genetic variation may impact our aroma perception, as does our diet.

It is common knowledge that our sense of smell is also closely linked to our sense of taste, and the joy of eating is impacted by how much we can smell. When our olfactory ability is diminished or absent it can have negative effects on mental health, sociability and well-being (Boesveldt & Parma, 2021; Pieniak et al., 2022).

Many years ago, a work colleague of mine had a fall which resulted in a blow to the head. As a result, she lost her sense of smell, and I remember her lamenting how food just wasn't the same anymore. How awful to be sat round a table with friends sharing a meal when they are all talking about how wonderful the food smells and tastes, all the while you smell nothing and your taste is impacted. The joy is sucked out of this experience and many others, so it is no wonder that there is a marked reduction in hedonic pleasures in life. A personal journey of smell loss is described eloquently in *On the Scent* (Totaro & Wainright, 2022). It is not surprising that there is an increased risk of depression if you have smell loss (Croy *et al.*, 2014; Eliyan *et al.*, 2021).

Aroma is linked to our being from very early on. I remember in the weeks before I had my daughter, I slept with a small toy popped down my nightshirt, because the baby books suggested she would then have the scent of me near her, when I was not. Odour is linked to many developmental aspects of human life, from the small baby being attracted to the aroma of a nursing breast (Boesveldt & Parma, 2021) to the child who gains comfort from the smell of something that reminds them of home. Even in the womb, the baby becomes attuned to the diet, environment, cosmetics and other substances that the mother may use, such as cigarettes via the amniotic fluid. Our responses to odours seem to be primed, from very early on in our existence, and as we continue to develop (Schaal, 2020).

Smell retains its importance as we move through the years. We recognize the smell of a lover's shirt or scarf, the perfume or aftershave of a loved one, the fragrance of our favourite food, plant or place. Aroma becomes entwined in our being, and it flows through our memories. Ask someone what one of their early aroma memories is and they will no doubt fall on a memory quite quickly. My grandparents' house had a distinct smell. Every summer we would visit South Devon for a fortnight and the aroma of the house was familiar and comforting. Decades later, I now experience a particular smell when I go to see my parents in their home. It is one that is hard to describe, it is unique to their home and very familiar. It is the smell of somewhere that is the closest thing to home, after my own home. The aroma is wrapped in my relationship with my parents and sister and the millions of memories that span the decades since my parents bought the house.

According to sociologist Schlinzig (2021), odour can create a sense of belonging and cohesion socially. In his qualitative research, he addressed the role of aroma for children and parents living in multiple homes. One child relayed how she had to get used to the smell in one parent's house being different from the other parent's house, and a mother told him how she had to wash her children's clothes when they came to visit as they didn't smell 'right' because their dad used different washing detergent. He notes that odours demarcate homes and territories.

He suggests that odorizing an object (that can be taken from place to place) allows for co-presence of the parent who is physically absent. So, just as we do this with babies (taking their favourite toy with them), perhaps we should pay more attention to enabling older children to still access the scent of another parent. I was talking to a friend about this chapter and as soon as I mentioned the associations we have with smell and places, she told me how her daughter says her mum's home smells different from her dad's home.

Aroma familiarity and preference may then be impacted by early memories, emotions, attachments, genetics, diet, learning and taste. Our memories of tastes and aroma can be intimately entwined (and we will explore how this works in the next chapter). One of my favourite biscuits is sultana and butter cookies from the British shop Marks & Spencer. My granny would buy them for summer picnics. They were expensive and a rare treat. Writing about them I can remember the buttery vanilla smell, the crunch of the biscuit and the chewy sultanas. My mouth instantly starts to water at the memory. The aroma, taste, texture and previous memory are interlaced in a rich dance. So much of our smell preference is socially constructed by our experiences and memories.

For me as an aromatherapist, aroma is clearly important. It's important to my clients too, even the ones who start coming to me because they are interested in the massage and not the aromatherapy. In nearly two decades, I have never had anyone come to me for a massage and not be happy to have essential oils added to the experience.

We must remember, however, that our sense of smell is often subjective. People will normally instinctively move towards an aroma that they like, often inhaling more deeply as they do so, or taking multiple sniffs, as if they are coming back for more. What elicits a positive reaction in one person does not necessarily do this for another. The best example I have of this is when I was working on a six-week project in a school for young people with special educational needs. I was working with a class of 16–17-year-olds, who were in the transition class, before they would move into adult care at the age of 18.

The school were amazing at providing a sensory experience, using sound, texture, colour and lighting in fun and creative ways. A previous member of staff was trained in aromatherapy but had since left, and I'd been asked to work with a small group of young people to provide an aromatic component. Working with the class and staff taught me so much. I had to think beyond my initial training and discover how I could offer them meaningful aromatherapy with my essential oils.

None of the young people could speak, one young man was deaf and partially blind, and for one young woman it was uncertain if she could hear or not. I also question if she was able to smell. All had extreme learning difficulties and they spent most of their day in a wheelchair due to physical disabilities. In the class I went into, staff would employ numerous bean bags and materials with different textures. The young people would be moved from their wheelchairs so they could either be supported by bean bags or move freely on the floor, depending on their wish.

One particular day, I was working with one young man who was deaf and partially blind. I was wafting a tissue near his nose with Roman chamomile (*Chamaemelum nobile/Anthemis nobilis*) essential oil on it, watching so I could gauge his reaction by observing his non-verbal clues. He did not react much to it, but out of the corner of my eye I saw a young woman turn quickly on the floor. She was crawling towards me, smiling and moaning, the noises she made getting louder and louder. I knew straight away that this would be the essential oil I would use for her when I worked with her later. In the meantime, I handed the tissue with the essential oil on it to her key worker who was nearby, so she could continue to access it and the joy it was bringing to her.

I always ask new clients about aromas that they like or dislike. Smell preference is important to aromatherapists, as we certainly have no wish to trigger someone with an essential oil, nor do we wish to use an aroma that simply offends someone. Lavender (*Lavandula angustifolia*) is often a smell that people really love or hate, and it is probably the essential oil that is most likely to be brought up as an example of something people don't like. In the UK, it is often viewed as an 'old person's' smell and may be negatively received, especially if there was an unpleasant older person in someone's life whose home smelt of it. Our memories are emotive and for most of us emotions are important. They also link intrinsically with physiological responses.

As I wrote about sultana and butter cookies earlier, my mouth watered (interestingly essential oils that remind us of food often elicit such a physical response and may make our mouths water, which is one of the reasons it is useful to smell citrus essential oils if someone has a dry mouth after cancer treatment). Thinking about the smell of the cookies not only made my mouth water, but it also gave me a sense of warmth, comfort and familiarity and I can almost conjure the aroma in my mind's nose. It is a secure, *safe* feeling. Feeling safe (as we will see later) is essential if we are to work with aroma and people who are looking to heal their trauma.

The preference for a vanilla type of aroma that Arshamian *et al.* (2022) noted really struck me, because a week before reading about the study, I'd been chatting to a friend who had told me that she always found comfort in the smell of vanilla. She went on to add that this was the smell of the reed diffuser in her counsellor's office.

She told me that her counsellor had worked hard to find an aroma that most people seemed to like and had settled on vanilla. Apparently, people would always comment on how nice her room smelt. Her counsellor was aware that no one can exclude a smell being a trigger or having a negative impact for someone. That said, there are times where we need a room to smell fresh.

When my friend smelt vanilla after this, it was a positive experience. Had she construed her sessions with her counsellors negatively, and had she felt unsafe in that environment, she may have felt differently about vanilla aromas. Alternatively, she may have had so many other positive attachments with the aroma (e.g. vanilla ice cream, vanilla cookies, perfumes) that this might have outridden any negative association. However, had she smelt vanilla during a traumatizing experience, or had she found her counselling retraumatizing, vanilla could have changed meaning for her and become a trigger.

We can also become used to odours over time (note I say odours and not triggers). Think about the individual who can no longer recognize that their house smells of cat litter trays because they live with this aroma all the time, or someone who has the smell of unwashed clothes or body odour on their person. When working with smell, we must also be careful that we don't over-habitualize someone to the aroma so that it no longer works for them (Herz, 2021), although this would probably only happen if there was daily exposure for a long period of time.

As an aromatherapist, I see the positive impact of aroma in my work all the time. If I can use an essential oil, hydrolat or CO_2 extract or a blend of these to produce a relaxing, safe, comfortable feeling for a client, then they can use this when they are with me, and I can create something for them to use elsewhere. The range of what I can offer is quite vast but is most likely to be an aroma stick inhaler (I find these very useful as they can be put in a pocket or handbag), a pulse point rollerball, a cream or lotion (either for the body or pulse points, heart centre or acupressure points), a diffuser blend or perhaps an aroma patch, or foot massage blend for someone who is bedbound.

As we will see in later chapters, essential oils, hydrolats and CO_2 extracts can be useful aromatic allies, as part of a longer-term holistic tool kit. They can be used in a multitude of settings. This should be done in a way that is individual (so as not to cause allergies or adverse reactions in others), informed and safe. They may be used before or during therapy, in hospital settings, rehabilitation centres, schools, refugee camps, aromatherapy consultation spaces, at home and more. Witnessing someone using them, especially as they work through their trauma, is an honour and a privilege.

Reflection points

- What are your earliest aroma memories?
- What is your favourite smell and why?

CHAPTER 2

How aroma works

If you are ambitious to found a new science, measure a smell.

Alexander Bell

The science of olfaction is complicated, and we know less about it than vision and hearing. Although it has advanced rapidly in the last three decades, there is still so much that we do not understand (Koyama & Heinbockel, 2020) and there are lots of misconceptions. For example, it is often assumed that as animals, human beings aren't very good at smelling. Maybe this is why our olfactory process is the 'Cinderella' of our senses (Barwich, 2020). Yet if our sense of smell is so poor, how can we smell and differentiate between tens of thousands (possibly even billions) of smells (Docter-Loeb, 2023)? Very small-scale research by Porter *et al.* (2007) suggests that humans may be able to scent track chocolate, which is a very surprising concept to most of us. So how does the complex process of smell work?

We smell through two mechanisms. The first is the most obvious one, where we use our nostrils. This is called orthonasal olfaction. The second is retronasal olfaction and this occurs when we eat food. As we place food in our mouth and chew it, it releases an aroma that goes from the back of our mouth up to our nose. It is thought that as much as 80% of the chemosensory information we receive when eating a meal comes through this pathway (Hummel & Podlesek, 2021).

Our senses of taste and smell are complexly linked, though we often forget this until we have a cold or something else diminishes, changes or stops our sense of smell. Do you remember those experiments at school where you were asked to pinch your nose and taste something and suddenly it didn't taste the same or was dulled? Let us consider how this complicated system works.

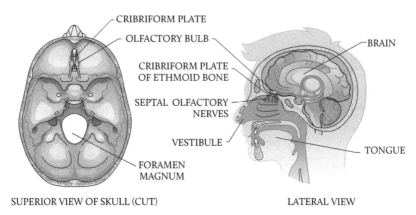

Figure 2.1: Olfactory system

When we inhale through our nose, tiny molecules enter the nasal cavity. As we pull air into our nose, structures inside our nose direct the airflow. They also cleverly filter it and warm it. One would assume that our nostrils smell things in the same way as each other but, as Barwich (2020) points out, this is not so. In fact, each nostril takes it in turn to vary the air flow speed by increasing swelling in the epithelium (a layer of tissue, sometimes referred to as mucosa). This allows us to smell a greater range of aromas.

When the molecules reach the olfactory epithelium, they bind to receptors. Signals are then created and passed to the brain through axons. These are little nerve fibres which pass from the olfactory epithelium, through the cribriform plate (a section of bone at the base of the skull), and into the olfactory bulb (there is a bulb for each nostril) (Fifth Sense, 2023). The olfactory bulb is a frontal lobe of the brain, and it sends signals to several other parts of the brain (Pieniak *et al.*, 2022), including the limbic system. The limbic system is one of the oldest parts of the brain (sometimes referred to as the reptilian brain). It includes the amygdala, thalamus, hippocampus and hypothalamus.

The limbic system is especially important here because it is connected to our memories, emotions, behaviours and fear responses. The hippocampus, for example, helps us form and retrieve memories, including autobiographical ones, whereas the amygdala helps us encode emotional memories and detect facial expressions and threat (Teicher & Samson, 2016). Understanding this, we can make sense of how memories and smell can be enmeshed and appreciate that smells can be a strong component of context-dependent memory (Hakim *et al.*, 2019).

Because of these fast and unconscious links within the brain, an aroma can illicit positive emotions and old memories, but it can also bring back negative ones, acting as a trigger for flashbacks and trauma responses (especially where there is PTSD).

Herz (2021) says that one of the reasons aroma triggers can be so incapacitating is that smells are invisible, and, in most instances, there is no prior warning. She reminds us that not only are smells handled in the same part of the brain that processes emotions, emotional memories and associations, but that this same part of the brain is also affected by PTSD. She tells us that the emotional brain will often process our response to smell before we have a chance to think it through cognitively with other parts of the brain. This explains why a smell that has become part of a trauma experience can be a trigger, even when it is experienced in different settings and contexts.

Herz (2021) also cites the work of Croy et al. (2010), whose research suggested that people with PTSD were quicker to respond to unpleasant smells (ones that were not triggers), and that the olfactory bulb volume was decreased in adults who had been maltreated as children. This is consistent with lots of other research that shows child abuse has been associated with changes in the brain's structure and function (Teicher & Samson, 2016).

Understanding that trauma in childhood impacts the olfactory system is crucial. The fact that smell is not routinely assessed in childhood (even though we check other senses such as hearing and sight) only serves to demonstrate how it is perceived as being less important. I think we should be checking whether children can smell as they grow up. This should be fundamental if a child has a trauma history. Lack of smell could be one more experience that they have not been able to own in comparison to their peers. This brings many challenges and feelings of 'otherness'.

Weiss et al. (2020) also suggest that smell screening early on in life could be beneficial because early smell training could reduce exposure to some of the negative implications of anosmia. Negative impacts of not being able to smell properly or losing one's sense of smell include depression, decreased enjoyment of food, difficulty with social interactions (such as eating a meal together, or avoiding social activities like wine tasting), issues with intimacy, fear of body odour or being unable to detect danger such as the smell of gas or smoke (Pieniak et al., 2022).

There has been a growing wealth of research in the scientific community that demonstrates the success of olfactory training, since Thomas

Hummel and his colleagues introduced this in 2009 (Pieniak *et al.*, 2022). After weeks of olfactory training, functional and structural changes in the brain have been observed, and optimum success appears to be with training that lasts around 32 weeks (Pieniak *et al.*, 2022). Olfactory training has been embraced within the aromatherapy community (especially after COVID-19), with colleagues also finding successful outcomes with participants individually and in classes (Galia, 2023), and in small-scale pilot groups (Mackereth & Carter, 2022).

It has often been assumed that if no olfactory bulb is present someone can't smell, yet Totaro and Wainwright (2022) state that at the time they were writing their book, Thomas Hummel was working with a woman who had no olfactory bulb. She had not been able to smell since birth, then in her twenties she began to smell. She could satisfactorily identify smells, even though she had not learned this as a child. This seemed astonishing. I then found a paper by Farruggia *et al.* (2022) where they suggested that maybe people without olfactory bulbs could smell using other, unknown pathways.

This possibility had been suggested earlier by Weiss *et al.* (2020). These researchers found two women who had no olfactory bulbs and by looking at an olfactory database of magnetic resonance imaging scans (MRIs) from over 1000 people, they discovered another three, possibly four women. All of these were women (women generally score better in smell tests), and all of them could smell!

The study also found a possible correlation between left-handedness and lack of olfactory bulbs, though much greater samples would be needed to verify this. They indicate that there could be a number of reasons that these women could still smell, even though there appeared to be no olfactory bulb present in MRI scans. One possible reason could be the migration of the olfactory bulb to a different brain location (although they postulate this would be likely to have been uncovered). They also suggest perhaps olfaction was being supported elsewhere in the cortex (previous studies with rodents who had had their olfactory bulbs removed had implied this might be the case), or that the olfactory bulb is simply too minute to be detected by the MRI.

Weiss *et al.* (2020) also note that maybe humans use the trigeminal nerve (this nerve controls facial nerves and helps us with biting and chewing) and other chemosensory nerve endings to make up for the loss of olfactory bulbs. Potentially we may compensate with different pathways. Interestingly, the trigeminal nerve also has a close relationship to the vagus nerve, as both are connected to a part of the brainstem called the ventral vagus complex, and we will explore this more in the next chapter.

Weiss *et al.* (2020) suggest that as many as 4.25% of left-handed women and 0.6% of women may be born without olfactory bulbs (or certainly not ones as we know them – as these can be seen on current MRI scans). However, it should be noted that a much greater sample size would be needed to verify this.

Researching this chapter was illuminating for me. It made me realize how little we understand about our sense of smell, how complicated it is and how little about smell the average person knows. For example, Rhind (2020) cites research that says that smells that enter the left nostril are accessed by the left side of the brain. Ones that enter the right nostril are accessed by the right side of the brain.

In the coming years, I expect we will understand far more, as science advances. Perhaps we will even gain a better understanding of whether the fear of a smell can be transmitted through generations.

Trials with rodents have already shown this may be possible. Debiec and Sullivan (2014) showed that mother rats transmitted their fear of an odour (peppermint) to their pups, impacting the pups' stress hormones and amygdala activity. In an experiment with mice, Dias and Ressler (2014) showed that mice that were conditioned to fear a smell, before even becoming pregnant, passed this fear of the same aroma to future generations. Even some of the neuroanatomy of the mice changed. While we have to understand that there are limitations to these studies (including the obvious fact that they are with rodents and not humans), the authors conclude that there is conceivable risk of intergenerational PTSD among humans, with behavioural and neuro-anatomical changes possible.

I am not aware of any human studies that demonstrate fear of a smell from generations before (and ethically conducting such a study would be more than a challenge); however, it has already been observed that babies born to mothers who experienced trauma when pregnant have altered hormone levels. An oft-cited example of this is babies born in the USA after 9/11 (van der Kolk, 2014). This is thought to be because of an in-utero reaction to the mother's trauma (many would say this resulted in direct trauma for the baby). Other research includes a small-scale study on mothers who were pregnant in Rwanda during the genocide, and descendants of Holocaust survivors. These studies suggest intergenerational trauma (sometimes also called generational or ancestral trauma), but as Youssef *et al.* (2018) point out, there are various limitations in the research and improved, larger-scale research would be helpful. While studies relating to smell triggers in future generations of humans may not be present (to my knowledge), it would seem plausible that such triggers could be passed into future generations.

How olfaction works is truly fascinating, especially in relation to our emotions, memories and fears. When I was a student aromatherapist many years ago, I was learning about the power of smell in relation to essential oils. Essential oils are naturally occurring fragrant substances that come from plant material. They are volatile which means they evaporate easily. They are derived through various methods (most commonly steam distillation, or in the case of citrus, most commonly expression) and we will explore this in more detail later in the book. To learn that these products could impact our mood and emotions because of the link between olfaction and parts of the brain was fascinating.

Olfaction is still an under-studied area that requires far more research, and there is much left to discover. In the next chapter, we will explore how the body and mind experience trauma and how this relates to what we know about smell.

Reflection points

- Have you discovered anything new about the process of olfaction?
- Which of your senses is most important to you and why?
- What can you do to develop your sense of smell?

CHAPTER 3

What is trauma?

Some distressing events are so extreme or intense that they over-whelm a person's ability to cope, resulting in lasting negative impact.

UK Trauma Council, 2023a

We cannot underestimate the effects of trauma on humanity, as it touches our lives on a micro and macro scale. Trauma is no longer thought to be about the event(s) itself. Instead, trauma is more commonly considered to be about the complex and diverse changes that take place within us, because of an overwhelming event or events or circumstances. These changes include unconscious bodily reactions (Levine, 1997; Maté, 2019; Porges & Porges, 2023; van der Kolk, 2014).

The effects of trauma can be long lasting and far reaching, affecting our physiological, mental, emotional, social and spiritual well-being, changing us biologically and potentially genetically (Porges & Porges, 2023). However trauma still often goes unrecognized and undiagnosed in society, even though as Bessel van der Kolk (2014) tells us, it leaves an imprint on someone's life.

People often shy away from talking about feelings (especially in the UK) and don't know how to manage the often-terrifying reactions they experience because of their trauma. Perhaps as a species we are so used to experiencing feelings of stress, that this stops us dealing with the pain of trauma even more. Levine (1997) suggests that trauma is such an integral part of the human experience that most people don't even recognize its presence.

From my research for this book and doing nearly two decades of aromatherapy and massage work, I am convinced that trauma plays more havoc with our bodies and minds than we are aware. As a student aromatherapist, I remember being told by my massage tutor that sometimes people's reactions to aromatherapy massage might surprise us. Occasionally, people may have a reaction to a trauma that their body had borne, and they may not even realize this memory had been stored in the body. Donna Robbins shares the example she gave to me when I was a student aromatherapist in Chapter 7. It stayed with me because I would see this play out on several occasions throughout my career.

There is a temptation to consider trauma as being experienced only by those living in war-torn countries, military personnel, or survivors of abuse, natural disasters or terrorist attacks. Yet this simply isn't the case. In fact, many trauma experts consider trauma to be part of human life (Levine, 1997). The UK government recognizes this diversity of experience, and says, 'Trauma results from an event, series of events or set of circumstances that is experienced by an individual as harmful or life threating' (UK Government 2022).

Some trauma types share different names, and definitions may differ between trauma experts and authors. This makes listing these types somewhat challenging. Some therapists (e.g. Hassan & Nettleton, 2023) say that anything that makes us feel unsafe and threatened can be traumatic, and that perhaps it is more realistic to think of life as being made up of various traumas, small traumas that we can manage or larger ones that are more problematic, overwhelming or devastating. Lewis *et al.* (2019) carried out a longitudinal study with over 2000 children. By the age the children were 18 years old, they found that almost one third had been exposed to at least one traumatic event and nearly 8% had experienced PTSD.

Trauma may be referred to as being acute, chronic or complex. Acute means it relates to one single event, such as being involved in an accident. Chronic means there is prolonged trauma that is repeated, for example living with someone who is violent, or being in combat. Complex relates to multiple, varied (and sometimes interrelated) traumas.

Trauma that happens within relationships is sometimes known as interpersonal trauma. This could include domestic abuse (intimate partner violence), child or elder abuse, or human trafficking (Lewis-O'Connor *et al.*, 2019).

In exploring what we understand by trauma, it is also necessary to understand that it may be experienced on a very individual level, within a family (this may go back generations), within culture, community or history, within wider society (and the structures therein) or collectively (en masse). To demonstrate the extent of trauma, I have listed some examples below. These are by no means a definitive list, but act as a starting point for considering the pervasiveness of trauma.

Individual trauma

Birth trauma, loss of a parent or close family member/friend, illness, physical injury (including accidents/falls, accidental poisoning), neglect, experiencing or witnessing violence or other abuse, rape and sexual assault, bullying, harassment, being homeless, medical/dental procedures, surgeries or prolonged immobilization (Levine 1997), being institutionalized, incarcerated or sectioned (Lewis-O'Connor *et al.*, 2019), miscarriage, still birth, lack of acceptance/being disowned by family and friends (e.g. in relation to sexuality or falling pregnant) and depression leading to suicide attempts are just a few examples of traumas that can touch someone's life.

It is now understood that babies and children's early experiences have a massive impact on their health. However, in the past, trauma in the uterus, attachment trauma and developmental trauma have sometimes been left out of conversations about trauma. In-utero trauma refers to trauma exposure before the baby is born (e.g. if the mother is taking drugs or is abused). Attachment trauma is a term used by some trauma specialists to refer to a poor emotional bond between a baby and mother (or father or other constant caregiver).

Developmental trauma refers to trauma happening in the first few years of a child's life, as the brain is developing. This is normally thought to be anywhere between the ages of birth to three or five, or even seven years old (although different experts have different ideas on this).

In 1998, Felitti *et al.* looked at the relationship between childhood abuse and household dysfunction and causes of health risk and ill-health in adults. Over 13,000 adults were surveyed and asked about whether they had experienced any of seven types of adverse childhood experiences (which we now abbreviate to 'ACEs'). These included physical, emotional or sexual abuse and living in a household where there were people who were substance users, or were violent, mentally ill or suicidal.

Over 50% of respondents had more than one ACE. As Felitti *et al.* (1998) found, ACEs correlated with multiple health risks later in life, so you will often hear the term ACE used in conjunction with trauma and links to poor health. This was seminal work in that it helped us understand the health implications of trauma in childhood. It also demonstrated that traumatic events in early childhood were far more common than suspected. However, if you are reading this and are concerned about health outcomes for you or someone else, please be reassured that such traumatic experiences do not mean you will become seriously ill. Much depends on other factors, including the psychological and social support and resources an individual has.

Although trauma may be experienced by the individual, it often extends beyond this. Families may have their own trauma histories that go back one or two generations, or ancestral trauma which goes back even further (and this in turn may relate to wider historical trauma and forms of oppression and violence).

Wider society

Trauma may also be shared within communities. It can also be cultural, historical, racial, or attached to sexuality or identity (Menakem, 2021).

Lewis-O'Connor *et al.* (2019) suggest that collective trauma can occur when circumstances are shared, for example in the case of homophobia. They also note it can be structural too and they point out that health-care institutions may unintentionally contribute to collective trauma through explicit and implicit bias in delivery of services. Other services, institutions and structures may also contribute to trauma (although there is the possibility to change this by developing services that are trauma informed, and we will explore this in Chapter 6).

Many minorities are also disproportionately affected by trauma. I recently read *Making It* by Jay Blades (2021). He details how his inno-cence was shattered when he went to secondary school, where he and another boy were routinely bullied and beaten because they didn't have white skin. He describes how there were certain places he couldn't go in London because of his skin colour and how he was regularly bundled into a police van as a teenager and young man for routine beatings from police.

Herz (2021) reminds us that in the USA, indigenous, African Amer-ican and Latin American populations are disproportionately impacted compared to non-Latino white people. In developing our understanding of trauma it is important to address these wider societal issues, even though it feels uncomfortable and difficult.

Asking people who are and have historically been impacted by trauma due to race to 'solve' the problem furthers negative narratives. It is therefore up to us all to honestly address our own feelings and bodily responses to racism, supremacy and colonialism. I found reading *My Grandmother's Hands* by Menakem (2021) an extremely helpful text and I would urge everyone to read it whatever their experience or skin colour.

Some authors (e.g. Menaken, 2021), suggest that trauma is rarely considered to be a collective human experience (if at all). COVID-19, I would argue, was a recent example of collective trauma. Yet instead of allowing people collectively to acknowledge, manage and grow from this, governments seem to have assumed that life should go back to normal. It is almost as if we can ignore the fact that it happened. Politically there may be reasons for this. Capitalism can only continue if we keep people working (and buying things). During COVID-19 we were told that the future would be called 'the new norm'. Yet many people see that the expectation of them is the same as it was before COVID-19, and sometimes even more is expected of them (especially by employers). The horrors that COVID-19 brought to our lives have been conveniently brushed away under the carpet for many. However, people seem angrier, more stressed and society more fractured than before.

Many of my clients say they feel differently after COVID-19. Some have struggled to return to the life they had before, and some avoid crowds and meeting new people. Perhaps this failure to acknowledge the trauma of the pandemic has created a state of cognitive dissonance. We are left with inner conflict.

We were given the message that we could not see people, and it wasn't safe to interact. We were locked down, separated and isolated, unable to visit the sick and vulnerable, unable to help or support the dying and not allowed to grieve in groups. Celebrating and congratulating the living through births, weddings and birthdays was off limits. Some people were left feeling alone, vulnerable, frightened and totally overwhelmed by this experience. Robbed of their time, social ability, support systems, freedom and norms. Going back to the pre-pandemic 'normal' has been impossible and highly difficult for some individuals. What they were told repeatedly and what they are now being told does not match up. Life now does not feel 'normal' or as it was pre-COVID. No wonder we are seeing higher levels of mental health, PTSD (Herz, 2021) and issues such as school refusal and anxiety in children and young people (Action for Sick Children, 2023).

Secondary (indirect or vicarious) trauma

Secondary trauma refers to trauma that is experienced as a direct result of working with, or being with, traumatized people. It is a potential occupational hazard that normally affects first responders (police, fire crew, medical staff etc.), social workers, therapists, workers in domestic violence projects, charity/crisis workers, legal workers and others involved in supporting them. It shares many of the symptoms of PTSD. Ellis and Knight (2022) note that the definitions are challenging, as terminology has developed over the years. They point out that in the earlier part of the 20th century, Freud was writing about counter transference, then Pearlman and McCann used the term 'vicarious traumatization', and in the 1990s Figley arrived at the term 'secondary' traumatic stress. I have also seen it called indirect trauma. While many professions provide advice, support and supervision and encourage self-care to guard against secondary trauma, many don't.

When I was discussing this with aromatherapist and herbalist Elizabeth Guthrie (who experienced secondary trauma as an emergency services dispatch handler), we talked about the language attached to the label. Secondary implies it is less than primary. The feelings and unconscious responses in our bodies, however, may remain the same. Trauma already brings shame, embarrassment and guilt. By calling it 'secondary' do we reinforce that? Ellis and Knight (2022) state that their qualitative interviews with service providers demonstrated that some had personal trauma histories (we will address the 'wounded healer' later in the book). This was useful as it allowed them to empathize. However, citing Ruiz-Junco (2017), the authors suggest it sometimes blurs a boundary between 'self' and 'other'.

Ellis and Knight (2022) found that previous trauma experience also makes people more vulnerable to secondary trauma, and many people they talked to had significant changes in their sense of self-agency. For example, participants struggled to trust people and they had intrusive images, overwhelming anxiety, uncontrollable crying, emotional outbursts, nightmares, insomnia, flashbacks to crime scenes, and a persistent sense of danger. It also impacted how emotionally available they were able to be with their families. Several were using drinking and smoking to 'numb' themselves. Ellis and Knight (2022) refer to secondary trauma as damage to the perception of 'self', noting that it may be produced by repeated empathic engagement.

In a previous work life, I attended and spoke at conferences aimed at medical staff. At first, I was truly amazed at the very dry, dark sense of humour that many of these professionals possessed, especially among those working on burns units. I soon realized that this is a necessary coping mechanism when you see such human suffering. In my clinical work, I have had many clients who are doctors, nurses, or are in the fire or police services. Many have intrusive images, nightmares or flashbacks regarding the things they have seen, heard and, of course, smelt.

I always remember an aromatherapy massage for a client who was a first responder. As I massaged, he started to recall someone he helped in his work. They had been badly maimed on the same part of the body I was currently working on. He mentioned that he would still think about the incident and dreamt about it occasionally. My feeling was that his body, his physiology, his very 'being' was remembering what it had seen. To some extent, perhaps he was merging himself and 'another', losing his 'self' in that moment, as Ellis and Knight (2022) suggested.

Disenfranchised trauma

Before researching this book, I had not heard of the term 'disenfranchised trauma', though I had heard the term connected to grief. It refers to trauma that is not, or cannot be, socially acknowledged. This may be partly due to the nature of the trauma. For example, if there is abuse or violence in the home, other family members are often not able to talk openly about this (it may even be avoided or denied). They may be impacted by what has happened but feel unable to seek support or talk about it.

Zoll and Davila (2023) provide a first-hand account of a sibling of a childhood sexual abuse survivor to illustrate this concept. The sibling talks about understanding that they were not supposed to talk about what had happened outside the counsellor's office, the guilt that this had happened to their sibling and the feeling that their family unit was damaged and no longer the same. This was compounded with other confusing feelings, such as how they felt about their father who was the abuser. Writing for an audience of social workers, Zoll and Davila (2023) recommend that victims of disenfranchised trauma and their families also need support, advocacy, assistance and acknowledgement, as they experience trauma, change and loss. The authors also recognize that intervention, information and therapy may also be helpful, and that the need for sibling support is in many cases likely to continue and heighten after trauma has been revealed.

As we have seen, there are so many trauma types – by recognizing these we can appreciate just how prevalent trauma is and start to realize the impact it has.

PTSD/Complex PTSD diagnosis

Not all people who are traumatized will have PTSD or complex PTSD, but their trauma experience(s) may still impact their life greatly. We therefore cannot limit discussions on trauma to PTSD. We also need to appreciate and understand that some people may have PTSD, but they will go undiagnosed. This may be because they do not seek a diagnosis, they do not have access to anyone who can help with a diagnosis, or their distress is not recognized by health professionals.

While it should be appreciated that you can have a trauma history but not have PTSD, we still need to explore and understand some of the challenges with PTSD diagnosis.

In the UK, National Institute for Health and Care Excellence (NICE) guidelines state that a PTSD diagnosis is normally made using the *Diagnostic and Statistical Manual of Mental Disorders (DSM-5)* or *International Classification of Diseases-11 (ICD-11)*. Both of these can be criticized for their definitions of trauma. The *DSM-5* definition states that trauma is a result of exposure to actual or threatened death, serious injury or sexual violence (UK Trauma Council, 2023b). It acknowledges that this exposure occurs when an individual directly experiences the traumatic event, witnesses it, or learns about it occurring to a close family member or friend, or that there is first-hand repeated or extreme exposure to aversive details of the traumatic event.

This definition disregards several categories of trauma (such as financial abuse or emotional control). The UK Trauma Council (2023b) also notes that it excludes trauma that comes from stigmatization, discrimination and violence perpetuated towards someone or groups of people due to sexual orientation, race, sex and other factors. It also doesn't seem to recognize foetal/in-utero trauma. As such I would say there is much room for improvement.

The World Health Organization (WHO) also produces the diagnostic criterion known as the *ICD-11*, which states that the traumatic event or events must have been 'extremely threatening'. The UK Trauma Council (2023b) criticizes this; after all, the word 'extremely' lends itself to subjectivity.

A PTSD diagnosis is normally given when multiple criteria are met. For example, with *DSM-5* an individual must experience at least one intrusive symptom from a list (including recurrent intrusive memories, nightmares, flashbacks/dissociative reactions (which could include passing out, or intense/prolonged distress after reminders, or physiological reactions to trauma-related stimuli). They must also be avoiding stimuli connected with the trauma and experience two or more negative changes to their mood. These should have either increased or begun after exposure to the trauma. The list includes inability to remember parts of the traumatic event, negative beliefs (about themselves or others), negative emotional states, reduced interest in activities that happened before the traumatic event, and a distorted sense of blame (either of themselves or others) for what happened. They are also required to have at least two changes in arousal and reactivity, which should have increased or began after the event. This list includes anger/irritability, self-destructive or reckless behaviour, hypervigilance, concentration issues, sleep problems and an exaggerated startle response. When the required number of symptoms are met, it is noted that they should be significantly distressing and impair function and be persistent for more than one month (National Institute for Health and Care Excellence, 2023a).

Another problem is that a diagnosis requires a memory of events (and memory can be affected by trauma). Some definitions also don't include complex PTSD, which is shocking (The Master Series on Trauma Conference, 2023) (we will look at how complex PTSD differs to PTSD in the next chapter). Birkmayer (2022) postulates that the exclusion of complex PTSD may be due to unconscious fear of the extent and impact of trauma in health. It also seems incredulous that trauma created for the baby in the womb, in the early years or through the generations is also ignored, especially as there seems to be growing evidence of transgenerational transmission of DNA methylations changes from parents to children (Youssef *et al.*, 2018).

A number of screening questionnaires may be used, such as the Trauma Screening Questionnaire, Impact of Events Scale-Revised, Davidson Trauma Scale and Post-traumatic Stress Disorder Checklist for DSM-5 (National Institute for Health and Care Excellence, 2023a).

I should point out that as individuals we do not always meet a diagnostic 'checklist'. Just because someone does not neatly mirror this list does not mean that they do not have trauma experience, nor does it mean that they should not receive or ask for help.

On a societal level, a diagnosis is often required by medical services to access treatment and satisfy medical insurance and treatment protocols, and may also be needed for budgets, forecasting, shaping future healthcare and more. Unfortunately, many people who experience trauma cannot afford to access necessary support and there is a danger that if you don't fit the diagnostic criteria, you might not get the help you need.

For many, a diagnosis can mean access to specialist support and understanding. It can mean people find help in working through the impact of their trauma. It may deepen individual understanding of physical symptoms, and how people feel about themselves and the world around them. Unfortunately, as with any diagnosis, some people occasionally experience negative effects (such as being 'labelled' or seen as a bundle of symptoms). Some people do not perceive themselves to be traumatized or they find that health or social care professionals involved in their care have not appreciated, understood or identified that their symptoms or difficulties relate to their trauma. Sadly, people do not always get the referrals and support that they need.

I have had several clients who have watched their life partner slowly die from terminal diseases. One of them said to me that for the medical professionals involved it was all about trying to 'make him better'. Close to the end, it switched to keeping him 'comfortable'. The indescribable trauma her husband, herself and her family went through was never properly acknowledged or addressed by medical staff. She was (and still is) traumatized by the experience. Yet according to some definitions this person would not be traumatized. Many trauma definitions can also be criticized as they focus solely on the individual. This is problematic as it doesn't encapsulate trauma due to societal problems, marginalization or prejudice.

It is truly hard to estimate how many people are impacted by trauma at any given time, as statistics are lacking and tend to *only* refer to those who have been diagnosed with PTSD. I would therefore argue that PTSD statistics are wildly unrepresentative of the level of trauma in society, and while they can be a helpful starting point, they should be read with this in mind.

Even though PTSD statistics are only recording a small percentage of actual human trauma, they are sobering reading. According to the UK charity PTSDUK (2023c), it is estimated that 50–70% of people will experience a traumatic event in their lifetime. Of these, approximately 20% will go on to develop PTSD.

It is important to understand that not everyone exposed to trauma will go on to experience PTSD. Several people may experience the same event, for example, but not all will have the same outcome. PTSD has several precipitating risk factors, including previous mental health issues, social support and sex. More women than men are diagnosed (Herz, 2021), though it is possible that this may be because more women than men seek diagnosis or support. It is thought that one in ten people are expected to experience PTSD at some point in their lifetime, and four in 100 people are expected to have PTSD at any given time (PTSDUK 2023c).

Other statistics from specific trauma experiences can be helpful in illuminating the potential prevalence. For example, in England and Wales, approximately one in four adult women and one in eighteen adult men are thought to have been raped or sexually assaulted as an adult (Rape Crisis, 2023).

In the UK, the NSPCC tell us that in 2023 there were 50,780 children named on child protection plans or registers (NSPCC, 2023). These children are just the tip of the iceberg as they are only the children who are known to be at risk. Many more children have experienced or are experiencing abuse. Statistics also look at the individual and this neglects wider-scale traumas that ripple through society and structures.

There is a lot to consider when we explore trauma. How we define, label, quantify, diagnose, support and help people heal from trauma is a complicated business. It may even be political at times, with political rhetoric and campaigns often adding further trauma. An example of the latter came to mind last year when I heard Bessel van der Kolk speak about ACEs at a conference. He mentioned how children's scores should not be recorded on their records because it has implications for health insurance (The Master Series on Trauma Conference, 2023). I wondered if this would have implications for certain schools and the wider community. It made me wonder how much statistics also get skewed by politics. If we really looked properly at trauma, the true picture would be beyond anything our crumbling UK welfare state can currently manage.

Reflection points

- Did you have any gaps in knowledge around types of trauma or terminology?

CHAPTER 4

What does trauma mean for the mind and body?

When we feel unsafe, our very senses change. Things taste, look, smell and sound different.

Porges & Porges, 2023, p.xix

Trauma has an extensive impact on our body, mind and soul. I have tried to divide symptoms into physical, psychological and behavioural issues to make it easier to read, though it is of course more complex than this. Below are the symptoms we could think about with regards to PTSD and complex PTSD (but please remember the experience of trauma is not limited to just those who have a diagnosis).

Physical sensations

- Trembling (especially if having a flashback)
- Sweating (especially if having a flashback)
- Racing heart (especially if having a flashback)
- Feeling spaced out/numb/detached from your body
- Feeling sick
- Feeling pain (e.g. headaches, chest pain, stomach aches)
- Tinnitus (PTSDUK, 2023a)
- Feeling dizzy
- Skin problems
- Hair loss
- Weight gain
- Digestive problems (e.g. irritable bowel syndrome)
- Difficulty building and maintaining muscle

- Cold hands and feet
- Fatigue
- Yawning
- Poor breathing patterns
- Allergies
- Problems with the immune system
- Muscular tightness, pain or physical limitations (Polatin 2020)
- Chronic pain (Lykkegaard Ravn & Andersen, 2020; Tesarz et al., 2020)

Psychological or behavioural aspects

- Intrusive or distressing thoughts or visual images
- Hypervigilance (feeling 'on edge')
- Sleep problems
- Nightmares
- Memory problems
- Being unable to remember details of the trauma
- Difficulty concentrating
- Emotional numbness
- Overwhelming negative feelings (e.g. shame, fear, guilt, anger)
- Feeling the need to be busy/hyperactivity
- Using alcohol or drugs to dampen, numb or avoid memories
- Self-destructive or risk-taking behaviours
- Feeling unsafe (with places, people etc.)
- Irritable or angry outbursts
- Aversion or reduced tolerance to sounds
- Avoiding potential triggers/reminders
- Difficulty feeling positive/happy emotions
- Difficulty trusting people (PTSDUK, 2023a)
- Difficulties with emotional regulation
- Feeling embarrassment, worthlessness
- Loss of interest in previous interests or job
- Difficulty making and maintaining relationships (Andrews et al., 2023)
- Difficulty making eye contact (Andrews et al., 2023)
- Avoidance behaviours, including agoraphobia, social anxiety and separation anxiety (Munyan, Neer & Beidel, 2016)
- Suicidal ideation (Blakey et al., 2018)

- Difficulty with peripersonal space (this may differ depending on whether someone is in a dorsal state or hypervigilant state) (Rabellino *et al.*, 2020).

Complex PTSD (C-PTSD)

Complex PTSD may include all the symptoms above, but it has additional, often more embedded aspects. It tends to be diagnosed in people who have had long-term trauma and/or experienced this early in their life. It often comes about when someone has been abused by someone who should have been a figure of trust, attachment and protection in their life. Examples might include someone who has been abused by a parent or other caregiver, or someone who was brought up in a cult or forced into sex work.

It can seriously impact how and if people are able to manage relationships, because the early attachment relationship often wasn't safe. Sometimes people totally avoid building relationships. Trusting others becomes an issue and it may be extremely difficult to form, sustain and keep healthy relationships.

The ability to do this may be further compounded by ongoing (normally constant) feelings of worthlessness, guilt and shame. Self-esteem can be crippled by complex trauma, and people often feel very different from everyone else. Emotional dysregulation may also be very extreme and constant, leading to a diagnosis of depression and suicidal thoughts, or even a preoccupation with getting revenge (PTSDUK, 2023a). PTSDUK (2023c) recognizes that it may also mean a loss of meaning in life, hope, value system or religion. Trauma can have a real impact on the soul.

As we see later in the chapter, complex PTSD also affects the brain in many ways. Some trauma specialists think that even particular mental health diagnoses, such as borderline personality disorder, may be misread and are in fact complex PTSD (e.g. Birkmayer, 2022; Fisher, 2023).

Other mental health diagnosis

People who have experienced trauma may also receive other mental health diagnosis – such as being depressed. Depression that results from a specific event, such as redundancy, losing your home or divorce, may be called reactive or situational depression. After birth trauma, a mother may be diagnosed as having post-natal depression. Depression and PTSD share some common symptoms.

Other behaviours – fawning and appeasement

In more recent years, other forms of reacting to trauma have also been identified. These include fawning, appeasement, dissociating, immobilization and freezing (we will address the latter three when we look at polyvagal theory later).

Fawning is people pleasing to diffuse conflict. It is about compliance, losing your identity to please another and reacting in the way someone else wants you to. For example, in a domestic abuse scenario, if a partner comes home from work angry, the abused partner may hurry to get them a beer, give them a comfy seat and do other things to try to placate them. Abused children may stay still and quiet and keep away from the abusive parent.

Appeasement, however, refers to situations where there is an attempt to co-regulate with the perpetrator of trauma, to maximize the chance to stay safe. Appeasement may occur when someone has been kidnapped, trafficked or is living with a violent partner.

Co-regulation is about mutual physiological regulation that comes about between people (Porges & Porges, 2023). Our words, tone of voice, behaviour, breathing, gestures and so on can all be used to soothe another person. An example of this would be a hostage talking calmly and softly to their kidnapper. Bailey *et al.* (2023) say appeasement is far better terminology than the previously used term 'Stockholm syndrome'. Stockholm syndrome has many deficits as a theory – it implies the traumatized individual wanted to be held captive, it insinuates the relationship is positive and it is set up from the point of view of the abuser. Bailey *et al.* (2023) say that this is confusing, diminishing and extremely unhelpful, especially to the traumatized survivor.

This perspective of the perpetrator having prominence to the detriment of the victim plays out time and time again in trauma. I was shocked to learn, for example, that old psychiatry manuals referred to father-daughter incest as being extremely rare (Herman, 2023) and not very harmful for the daughter (van der Kolk, 2014). They are written from the perspective of the perpetrator and not the victim and are layered in misogyny and patriarchy. Similarly, the criminal justice system serves to protect the person accused of rape ('innocent until proven guilty') and yet the rape victim is put through a retraumatizing trial, on top of invasive physical examinations, police interviews and so on. Herman (2023) cites Campbell *et al.* (2001) who describe the trial process as a 'second rape'. In the USA, it is thought that only between 1 and 5% of all rapes are prosecuted, with fewer than 5% resulting in a guilty plea or conviction (Herman, 2023).

Fawning and appeasement can occur in relation to many different traumas, not just interpersonal trauma. At an international trauma conference in 2023, Linda Thai discussed how people of colour sometimes feel they must fawn and appease white people's guilt for their ancestors' oppressive and brutal actions, which can be exhausting (The Master Series on Trauma Conference, 2023).

Long-term health issues

Repeated trauma may also be referred to as 'toxic stress'. This refers to excessive or prolonged activation of stress responses in the body (Lewis-O'Connor *et al.*, 2019).

Many trauma experts who have been physicians for decades have noticed how clients with trauma histories have a higher propensity to have long-term medical conditions such as Lupus or rheumatoid arthritis (Maté, 2019). Science is now pointing towards a relationship between our neurological, endocrine, immune, autonomic, inflammatory and metabolic processes and trauma (Katrinli *et al.*, 2022; Lewis-O'Connor *et al.*, 2019; Porges, 2009; van der Kolk, 2014).

These long-term health problems, such as irritable bowel syndrome, gastric reflux, fibromyalgia, chronic fatigue, various cardiac issues or migraines (Levine, 2018), can impact health across the lifespan. Felitti *et al.* (1998) found a graded relationship between the number of ACEs and ischemic heart disease, cancer, chronic lung disease, skeletal fractures and liver disease. They also found an increased health risk of suicide attempts, depression, obesity, alcoholism, drug abuse, smoking, sexual partners and sexually transmitted diseases.

Lewis-O'Connor *et al.* (2019) cite Coker *et al.* (2002), who found an increased risk of chronic disease and depressive symptoms, chronic mental illness and substance addiction among people who had experienced intimate person violence. When our bodies are under extreme stress, Polatin (2020) reminds us that our energy goes towards protection, rather than finding a place of homeostasis, leaving us vulnerable to illness. Trauma can also make us more sensitive to pain (e.g. Lykkegaard Ravn & Andersen, 2020; Tesarz *et al.*, 2020).

Some of the research around the impact on the body throws up conflicting results. For example, Murphy *et al.* (2022) propose that early childhood trauma such as abuse that occurs while the brain is developing may influence the hypothalamic-pituitary-adrenal (HPA) axis (previous research showed conflicting results as to whether the HPA axis was affected). The age and sub-type of trauma, they determined, was important.

When we consider the health implications of trauma, Lewis-O'Connor *et al.* (2019) remind us that trauma experiences may also mean that people avoid using healthcare services in the first place (and we will address this more in a later chapter on trauma-informed care). Service use avoidance may further exacerbate medical conditions and long-term illness, and result in poorer outcomes.

During my research, my interviews with other aromatherapists reminded me continually how trauma shows up for different people in different ways, and how personal the experience is.

On the one hand, we need to understand the range of symptoms people experience so we can recognize trauma and respond to it, but on the other hand, using the term 'disorder' (as in PTSD/C-PTSD) can sometimes be negative for people. As everyone is unique, some people may experience symptoms that aren't even discussed in this chapter in relation to their trauma.

These symptoms are an adaption to overwhelming circumstances (Hassan & Nettleton, 2023). They have occurred to keep us safe and help us survive the trauma. The difficulty is that our body doesn't know that it no longer needs this adaption and people continue to experience awful symptoms that often impede everyday life. As trauma expert Babette Rothschild (2000) tells us, 'The body remembers'.

The autonomic nervous system

We cannot address the topic of trauma without looking at the role of the autonomic nervous system (ANS). Within the ANS we have the parasympathetic nervous system and the sympathetic nervous system.

Most people have heard of the sympathetic nervous system. It is what enables us to be active and mobilized. We often hear the term 'flight or fight' mode. This relates to the sympathetic nervous system and how our body reacts to perceived threat. Either we flee and run away, or we stay with the threat and fight. When our flight and fight activation is consistently engaged/over activated we can become hyper aroused. This can happen due to trauma exposure. Hyperarousal may display in numerous ways, such as fast heart rate, feeling panicky, hypervigilance, being easily startled, irritability, anger or rage.

In contrast, the parasympathetic system is sometimes referred to as the 'rest and digest' state, as it does many things we associate with relaxing, such as helping us with sleep, digestion or lowering our heart rate. Stephen Porges critiques this way of looking at the ANS as it assumes that we are always in one state or the other (Porges & Porges, 2023).

Therapists around the globe have known for some time that when faced with trauma, many people do something that is not 'flight' or 'fight.' Instead, they immobilize and are involuntarily and physically unable to flee or fight. An example is someone 'freezing' when attacked. The body, to survive, almost shuts down. This is common in sexual assault. In some instances, people might shut down completely and pass out (this is sometimes referred to as 'flop' to distinguish it from freeze).

We see this freezing and immobilization happen in nature. If a cat catches a mouse and the mouse freezes, the cat might get bored or lose interest. The mouse may then be left alone, with the possibility of a later escape. It is an unconscious, involuntary and useful survival technique and it extends to humans.

People who have experienced sexual assault are sometimes asked why they did not fight or run away. Porges and Porges (2023) point out that this is based on assumptions of what the other person thinks they would do, even when they have no personal experience. When people make comments like this, they are thinking with the problem-solving part of their brain, but when we are in survival mode, we are in fact thinking with the oldest, reptilian part of our brain. We are just focused on survival.

This myth that the body only goes into flight or fight mode and that someone can choose to fight or flee is unhelpful and can be hugely detrimental. It can also be incredibly shaming because it implies choice. In such moments, the bodily response is involuntary. This has been confirmed by trauma experts and polyvagal theory (e.g. Herman, 2023; Porges & Porges, 2023). It is crucial to understand this and if you are reading this book and have ever been in a state where you could not flee or fight, know that your body responded in this way to keep you safe.

Therapists and trauma workers also see dissociation, where someone feels as if they are not in their body, or they are separating off. Such behaviours are often described as states of hypoarousal and again they occur as an instinctive survival strategy that supports the person so they can manage such a horrific and overwhelming experience.

Polyvagal theory (PVT)

Porges developed a new theory called polyvagal theory in the 1990s. This incorporated neuroanatomy and neurophysiology, gave a new insight on the working of the ANS and theorized that feeling safe came from inside the body, and that social connection was important (Porges, 2009, 2022).

At this time, other trauma workers were noting that there was a need to work with what people were experiencing in their bodies (and not rely on only working through traumatic memories). Work was developing in somatics, with Peter Levine writing *Waking the Tiger* in 1997. Therapists and psychiatrists were also noticing that talking therapies alone were not always working for people who were traumatized and that rehashing traumatic memories could sometimes retraumatize people (van der Kolk, 2014).

So how was polyvagal theory useful in addressing trauma? Porges told us that we need to go beyond looking at just 'flight and fight' within the sympathetic nervous system, and that we needed to address the role of the vagus nerve within the ANS.

The vagus nerve is a cranial nerve that begins in the brainstem and goes into the torso, linking to many parts of the body (hence the term vagus, which means wandering in Latin).

Earlier I mentioned the parasympathetic nervous system. Its primary neural pathways are vagal (of the vagus nerve). The majority (about 80%) of the messages sent through this nerve are from the body up to the brain, so messages from organs and visceral sensations are being communicated to the brain from the body.

Porges postulated that the body wants to feel safe and socially connected. The ventral (front) part of the vagal nerve enables this, yet it only occurs in modern mammals, including humans. It is sometimes called the modern vagus. It is restorative for the body and impacts positive social connection, through its connection to things like facial and vocal features.

Trauma can disrupt the (modern) ventral vagal state, meaning we no longer feel safe and socially connected and cannot (or find it difficult to) co-regulate. Co-regulation is important because it allows us to sense and work in harmony with others to enable mutual feelings of safety and social connection. For instance, if someone has a panic attack, we can talk calmly and quietly and model a good breathing pattern, and as they fall into this with us, we are co-regulating.

The dorsal vagal system differs to the modern ventral vagal state, as it is much more ancient. It is found in reptiles as well as mammals and it plugs into the back of the brainstem. It is this 'old' dorsal vagal system that is thought to facilitate the freeze (immobilizing) response.

So, Porges extended our thinking on the ANS by suggesting that we go beyond traditional thinking on the parasympathetic and sympathetic nervous systems, and that we also consider the role of vagus nerve and its ventral and dorsal pathways. In doing so, we would appreciate more fully how our nervous system and entire body responds to and is altered by how safe we do, or don't, feel (Porges & Porges, 2023).

By using the term 'neuroception' Porges explained how the autonomic nervous system within our body responds in a totally unconscious way. This is very different to perception, which is a cognitive process.

What was exciting for me, as an aromatherapist and body worker, was that it explained so much of what I saw in terms of bodily reactions in people, long-term medical conditions and some of the things I had experienced or heard about in my former career.

Initially, there were some criticisms of polyvagal theory (such as a lack of evidence), but trauma workers, therapists and psychiatrists and other trauma experts were finding that the theory fitted their experience of working with people who had experienced trauma. There are many similarities and overlaps between the work of several trauma authors at this time (including Peter Levine, Bessel van der Kolk and Gabor Maté).

The impact of trauma on the brain

Research using MRIs and studying people with a formal PTSD diagnosis is still relatively young. However, studies have demonstrated that changes in communication in the brain occur as a result of trauma (Teicher & Samson, 2016; PTSDUK, 2023b). We have already explored how emotions and memories are entwined, with smells being a strong component of context-dependent memory (Hakim *et al.*, 2019). There is potential for the brain to be reactive to an aroma it associates with previous trauma, even when the context has changed, because sadly trauma can literally change the body, the mind and the brain (van der Kolk, 2014).

We saw earlier how the hippocampus (part of the limbic system) helps us form and retrieve memories, including autobiographical ones; however, this part of the brain is vulnerable to damage from cortisol, which we know there can be an excess of under stress. The amygdala, which helps us encode emotional memories and detect facial expressions and threat, is also prone to change due to trauma, especially in early childhood (Teicher & Samson, 2016).

However, research has sometimes confusingly thrown up differing results in these brain changes. Zilcha-Mano *et al.* (2022) note that some research seems to show that patients who have PTSD have smaller hippocampus volume, while different studies show they have not. Similarly, some findings show a reduced amygdala size, while others found a larger size. Why is this the case?

Zilcha-Mano *et al.* (2022) suggest more longitudinal studies, larger sample sizes, tighter control conditions between MRI sites and more diversity among participants are needed in the research, but it is startling to see how much change can occur.

Teicher and Samson (2016) propose that several factors may be at play in these differing results. Variables include the type of trauma, age at exposure to trauma, age at MRI, sex (with the protective effect of oestrogen being one hypothesis for reduced volume of the hippocampus in men but not women), and the time period between exposure to trauma and being able to observe changes in the brain. They point to various research papers that imply that early separation stress has a larger effect on synaptic density in the hippocampus than the prefrontal cortex, whereas adolescent stress has a bigger impact on the prefrontal cortex than the hippocampus. They even cite Luby *et al.* (2013), who conducted a longitudinal study and found that poverty influenced volume of the left hippocampus, and supportive-hostile parenting influenced the right (Teicher & Samson, 2016).

In an attempt to explore some of these different findings regarding brain structure that researchers were noting, Jeong *et al.* (2021) carried out a large-scale study of 9270 nine- and ten-year-olds. They were trying to eliminate some of the previous research problems related to differing ages or small sample size. They also aimed to control for income and parents' education (presumably attempting to rule out social economic status as a factor). The results still showed that trauma affected the brain structures, with thinning and thickening in different areas and reduced volume in the right amygdala and right putamen. The authors, like so many others, concluded that childhood trauma may indeed be a risk factor for the developing brain.

In adults, when looking at peripersonal space and bodily self-consciousness, Rabellino *et al.* (2020) note that many parts of the brain are impacted by trauma, including the prefrontal cortex, intraparietal sulcus, putamen, supramarginal gyrus, postcentral gyrus, cerebellum, insula and vestibular system, and this was impacting how people felt about peripersonal space and how bodily self-conscious they were.

Andrews *et al.* (2023) addressed social cognition processes in adults with PTSD by observing differences in the brain activity of adults with

PTSD versus a control group. They exposed the participant to a neutral memory and then asked them to view an avatar's face (both side on and face on, with direct eye contact). Then the participant was exposed to the trauma memory and then the avatar's face again, in the same manner. Both times the participants were asked to identify the emotion of the avatar and how they felt towards the avatar. While there are possible downfalls of this study (e.g. results could be skewed by the gender/appearance/similarity of the avatar to someone they know, and it was small-scale research), the results were illuminating. Participants who had PTSD had greater activation in areas such as temporoparietal junction, left cerebellum crus II and right MSFG than the control group. This combination of differences, the researchers pointed out, resulted in different social cognition processes, and impacted how the group who had PTSD wanted to react when confronted with eye contact and how they felt themselves (Andrews *et al.*, 2023).

According to Zilcha-Mano *et al.* (2022), it is even possible that parts of the brain change just by exposure to trauma (regardless of whether someone has been diagnosed with PTSD or not).

A study by Zhu *et al.* (2022) found that the participants with PTSD could complete the same task as someone else who had no trauma exposure, but, when they felt threatened, they found the task more difficult. Intriguingly, the participants' MRIs showed there was less signalling between the hippocampus and the salience network. The salience network is linked to learning and survival. There was also reduced signalling between the amygdala and the default mode network (this part of the brain activates when someone isn't focused on the outside world, for example when we go onto 'auto' pilot on a journey because we are so used to doing the route).

In an interview, Suarez-Jimenez sums this up for the lay person by saying it suggests that emotions overtake the ability to distinguish between safety, danger and reward, and it would appear that there is a bias towards danger (Smith Hayduk, 2022). This is fascinating because as soon as I read this, I was mindful of *feeling* safe as being the main tenet of polyvagal theory.

Further research Suarez-Jimenez has been involved in also suggests that some people can possibly work around the change that happens in the brain. This feels promising and hopeful (Zhu *et al.*, 2022).

Our brains are intricate, complicated structures, but it is clear through numerous studies and MRIs that trauma does indeed impact the brain, when we look at research comparing people with PTSD to people without PTSD. In some instances, it creates excessive communication between different parts of the brain. In other instances, communication may be diminished, and even the volume of parts of the brain can be changed. People who have complex PTSD because of childhood trauma have differing MRI results, as the brain was developing when the trauma occurred. There is still more to discover, but by understanding this we can appreciate how difficult trauma makes people's lives and why some of the symptoms of trauma occur. It is hoped that through such work we can also develop a better understanding of how to support people in the future.

Getting treatment and help

Access to support for trauma around the world differs. It is worth exploring what is available in your country.

Trauma expert van der Kolk (2014) states that three routes seem to be available: top down (e.g. connecting with others, talking about it and processing it), bottom up (exploring bodily reactions and enabling the body to have reactions that differ to the helplessness, anger, immobility and so on experienced within the body as a result of trauma) and medication that acts on the hypersensitivity the brain experiences, or other technologies that help the brain classify information. The range of support and help available might include talking therapies, support groups, psychiatry, drama, movement or art therapy or complementary therapies.

In the UK, the first line of treatment for trauma within our National Health Service (NHS) is normally trauma-informed cognitive behavioural therapy (CBT) and eye movement desensitization processing (EMDR) (National Institute for Health and Care Excellence 2023b). This may be offered even if you don't meet diagnostic criteria for PTSD. Exposure therapy that includes aroma is being trialled in the USA (more on this later in this chapter), and medication (including antidepressants) may also be offered.

For aromatherapists like myself, it is important to know if someone is taking prescription medication, as there may be interactions between some essential oils and medication.

It is also important that we are aware of new and upcoming treatments, such as the use of psychedelics (such as MDMA or ketamine) alongside talking therapy. At a 2023 international trauma conference in the UK, Bessel van der Kolk reported that these are showing 'stunning promise' for trauma work, if used safely and correctly (The Master Series on Trauma Conference, 2023). There is, however, much more research required.

With advancements in science (such as brain scans and new theories like polyvagal theory), we now appreciate the complexity of trauma for humanity. We are finally realizing the consequences of trauma both for the individual, and wider society, but we still have a long way to go. Next, we will look at how aroma and trauma intersect – a notion that is often forgotten but warrants further study.

Reflection points

- What have you learned about the impact of trauma on the brain and the body?

CHAPTER 5

The intersection of aroma and trauma

We have seen how smell can be impacted by the experience of trauma. In cases of developmental trauma, we have seen how the development of children's brains is affected and that this can even lead to an absence of olfaction (Herz, 2021). If olfaction from the womb onwards provides scaffolding for learning throughout different developmental aspects of childhood and adolescence (Schaal *et al.*, 2020), we can see how this might have many implications for those whose smell is impacted by trauma. Some research has proposed that for some individuals who experience different types of trauma, sense of smell might even be heightened in some circumstances (Herz, 2021).

Of course, we also know that smells can be triggers. War veterans will talk about the stench of diesel, sand, burning hair, burning flesh, plastic (Lewis & Ossola, 2023) or blood (Cortese, Leslie & Uhde, 2015) for example. The smell of alcohol (Lewis & Ossola, 2023) or aftershave/cologne (Guthrie, 2023) can be a common trigger for people who have experienced sexual abuse or domestic violence.

Clinical aromatherapist Cynthia Tamlyn and I talked about aroma and triggers when I interviewed her for this book. She pointed out how important it is to ask about smell preferences and dislikes on our intake (consultation) forms. For example, she mentioned that Hops essential oil reminded her of beer. The aroma of alcohol can be triggering for some people. Elizabeth Guthrie (2023) writes that she was reminded by someone that woody essential oils can sometimes be reminiscent of cologne, which some people may also need to avoid.

Smelling a particular aroma again (even years later) may generate an unconscious trauma response. This is because the older part of the brain that is involved in smell is connected to emotions and memories and it is telling the person, 'There is that smell again. I don't feel safe.' It is innocently picking up on the scent and signalling threat, even though the context of the aroma is different.

The person may *be safe* (because the circumstances are different), but the brain doesn't make this distinction (Porges & Porges, 2023). Instead, the brain responds to the smell as a threat to be feared, employing a survival response in return that can show up in the mind, body and behaviours in many ways, and even trigger flashbacks. Cortese *et al.* (2015) note that these 'odour threats' are very specific to the individual.

Aroma triggers are instinctual, unconscious, fast and often terrifying, and it is important to note that individuals can't simply rationalize the smell as being safe. In MRIs, we have seen that the prefrontal cortex, (the newest, more progressive, human part of the brain that helps us problem solve and rationalize) shows less activity in people with PTSD. It is less engaged. Some trauma researchers and experts state that this is possibly one of the reasons that top-down ways of working (top referring to head, so for example talking therapies such as CBT) aren't always as successful as bottom up (which is more body-centred trauma healing) (van der Kolk, 2014).

In her autobiography about her nursing career, Christie Watson (2018) mentions how colleagues could be impacted by PTSD. She talks of how she starts to feel nothing and finds herself 'closing down'. She recalls an incident when two children had been brought into paediatric intensive care after being in a house fire. Watson recalls washing the girl's hair because all that could be smelt was the stench of smoke. She describes the ward as smelling of fire, replacing the normal aroma of antiseptic. She says patients like this, and the smell of smoke, will stay with her forever.

The impact of odour as a memory and a trigger should never be taken lightly. It can be debilitating (Herz, 2021) and it can be extensive. Hinton *et al.* (2004) found that out of 100 Cambodian refugees, 45% had suffered an odour-triggered panic attack in the previous month. That is a lot of people experiencing odour triggers.

Cortese *et al.* (2015) illustrate that while smells are normally processed through the olfactory pathway, they may also activate the trigeminal pathway causing irritating sensations such as burning or stinging. An example of this is ammonia.

Many years ago, one evening, I worked on someone who struggled to care for himself properly. He must have had some urine on his clothes. The smell was very strong, and even though I was using an essential oil blend to massage his lower legs and feet, the urine odour was all I could smell. It was intense and stung my nostrils. Afterwards, I inhaled Lemon essential oil and even tried Peppermint (*Mentha x piperita*) in my attempt to banish the smell but nothing worked.

I went home, but still it stayed, as strong as ever. I gave up, showered and went to bed. Thankfully, in the morning it had gone. The sensation in the nose, alongside the smell, cannot be underestimated. Unfortunately, in war or disaster zones certain smells like burning or certain gases can last for hours, days or weeks. Where there have been floods, the smell of dampness, mould and things rotting can take hold. Veterans have spoken about smells like burning being in their clothes and hair, making them cough (Lewis & Ossola, 2023).

New ways of thinking...

Cortese *et al.* (2015) cite a few research teams who have suggested that olfactory perception can be potentiated by trigeminal activation (Bensafi *et al.*, 2007; Hummel & Livermore, 2002; Moessnang *et al.*, 2013). They postulate that aromas with strong trigeminal properties may be more likely to become a conditioned odour threat (Cortese *et al.*, 2015). This got me thinking: remember we saw in polyvagal theory how the vagus nerve is closely linked to the trigeminal nerve, as both are housed in the ventral vagus centre (Porges & Porges, 2023)? When a smell has a physical impact on the nose or throat, does this somatic element mean the odour can be felt as well as smelt? If so, why aren't we addressing this?

Extending this thought, might it be tasted too? We know people talk of smells lingering (e.g. burning plastics or smoke) and perhaps if people are eating or drinking while smelling this horrific aroma are they also experiencing the aroma both orthonasally and retronasally? And what does this then mean for their body and their trauma?

Physiologically, smells have the capability to be experienced in different, yet highly connected, ways. Our bodies even have olfactory receptors in places other than our olfactory system. They are also expressed in the skin, gastrointestinal system, heart and kidneys and although they don't sense odours like our olfaction system does, they are involved in chemical reactions, adjusting blood pressure and stimulating hormones and enzymes (Koyama & Heinbockel, 2020). In essence, odours can potentially affect how we feel regardless of our olfaction system and the link between our olfactory bulb and our brain.

While smell can be a sense by itself, perhaps we should not separate it from its relationship to soma. Maybe we should explore the relationship and link to the trigeminal nerve in more depth.

Can olfaction be further woven into theories that help us understand trauma and its relationship with our body (such as polyvagal theory)?

Some researchers have found they can harness an aroma that is triggering and use it to benefit people struggling with PTSD. Exposure therapy is a form of therapy whereby people are exposed to their fear/previous experience in a graduated manner, with the aim of gaining more control over their memories (Lewis & Ossola, 2023).

Recently, researchers have started using virtual reality (VR) technology as a way of conducting exposure therapy. Virtual reality exposure therapy has harnessed highly specific, individualized aromas, sounds and visuals and seems to yield promising results. Herz (2021), notes that it even has potential to reduce or stop people getting PTSD if they are habitualized before going into specific environments like war zones.

In the past, exposure therapy was often used for phobias, but VR has made it possible to recreate other experiences, such as an explosion for a war veteran. Deborah Beidel, a clinical psychologist and executive director for UCF Restores, explains that in the clinical research centre for PTSD that she heads up, they have trialled this with first responders and survivors of sexual assault as well as veterans. In some instances where visuals aren't possible, they have been able to use sound and smells with just as effective results (Lewis & Ossola, 2023). Using VR in this manner is still in its infancy, but it is fascinating to see its potential.

As an aromatherapist, I ask about negative associations with smells and any triggers on my consultation (intake) forms. I never used to use the word trigger, but because it is now more readily understood, I do. I think it shows how seriously I take the issue of trauma and it reminds people how important their sense of smell is. I do not currently ask about people's ability to smell; however, I am now wondering if I should.

It is important that we know about triggers or trauma histories so we can avoid certain essential oils. If you know the context of someone's trauma it may help to distinguish what not to use. Essential oils such as Frankincense (*Boswellia carteri*), Copal santo (*Bursera copallifera*) and Breau branco/Brazilian frankincense (*Protium heptaphyllum*), to my mind have a slightly fuel-like odour. Given that fuel can be a smell trigger, especially with those who have worked in combat zones, or experienced aviation or automobile accidents, it would be worth avoiding these, especially in single use. Sometimes we do not have this information, and people do not know that an aroma will be a trigger, but we can do our best with the information we have.

The mental health charity Mind (2016) produced an excellent video (available on YouTube) that explores four people talking about their experience of dissociation. One of the group notes how she sometimes uses incense, Lavender (*Lavandula angustifolia*; possibly the essential oil but it is not clear) or a hand cream with a strong smell if she is going out and is worried about dissociation (or 'drifting off' as she says). The aroma, she says, brings her back to the present.

I have seen many instances of how aroma can be used in a positive way – to ground and anchor someone in the current moment; to help someone feel calm and safe enough so they are able to have something like a medical procedure that was previously utterly terrifying for them.

I have a client who had a panic attack when she went for an MRI. She told me, 'It was just horrendous.' When she mentioned she would need another MRI, she said she was absolutely dreading it. I told her I could give her something to help her with this. I made her a pulse point rollerball, with 10ml of Sweet almond oil, and 3 drops of pre-diluted Rose essential oil (this was from a 10ml bottle containing 90% Jojoba oil and 10% of *Rosa damascena*), 3 drops of Neroli (*Citrus x aurantium*), 2 drops of Copaiba (*Copaifera officinalis*) balsam (not the essential oil), 2 drops of Geranium (*Pelargonium x asperum*), 1 drop of Cedarwood atlas (*Cedrus atlantica*).

I told her to apply it to her wrists, her neck, behind her ears and on CV17 (an acupressure point which I have found very helpful for clients). I gave her a colour and breath relaxation exercise to do, and suggested she practise this several times, using her pulse point rollerball. This blend was familiar to her, as these were essential oils she has been exposed to before in her aromatherapy massages.

Interestingly, this client has quite a poor sense of smell and commented that her sinuses felt very blocked on the day. At this point I could have chosen a different approach and might have gone with a blend that would help with the sinuses, but my aim was to support her with her anxiety and fear, to prevent a panic attack so the procedure could be carried out. The blend I gave her would help her feel comforted, relaxed and safer, and, importantly, it was a familiar aroma that reminded her of a time she was relaxed, having her aromatherapy massages. I was thrilled to get a message later that day, to say that the MRI had happened successfully.

There are several other aromatherapists using aromatherapy to support people who struggle with medical procedures. For example, Mackereth, Carter and Maycock (2023) give wonderful examples of their ability to use aromatherapy to support people who have needle phobia.

Why are essential oils particularly useful when working with trauma and aroma?

We have already seen that the process of olfaction and the limbic part of our brain are closely linked, meaning certain smells that relate to positive memories can be emotionally supportive. Many parts of the brain may also be positively impacted by smelling essential oils. For example, Birkmayer (2022) notes that the default network mode (part of the brain involved in introspective thinking, rumination, self-focus, mental time travel and so on) can be impacted by PTSD. He cites Karunanayka *et al.* (2017), who say that through olfaction positive changes for the default network mode can occur.

Science has been able to show for some time that essential oils can be extremely useful because of their naturally occurring chemical makeup. They have many useful properties such as being antidepressant, anxiolytic, sedative and cognitive enhancing (Rhind, 2020). Clinical studies have shown that essential oil use can effect changes in blood pressure, heart rate, cortisol levels, brain waves and feelings of calm or alertness (Lizarrange-Valderrama, 2021). Crucially, essential oils have the ability to impact our nervous system (Langley-Brady *et al.*, 2023).

Mortensen (2023) reminds us that changing heart rate variability is often deemed to be a measure of vagus nerve activity, so knowing that certain essential oils can do this can be very helpful. Applying polyvagal theory, we can see the potential for aromatherapy to help us enter a ventral (modern) vagal state and reach homeostasis.

When used in a dermal application, the essential oils are absorbed into the body, but the person also benefits from smelling the essential oil. If one is to follow polyvagal theory, there are parts of the body that may benefit from massage, using an aromatherapy blend including the neck and ears. Mortensen (2023) cites Meier *et al.* (2020), who indicate that targeted neck massage in the area between the trapezius and sternocleidomastoid muscles may be helpful. Alternatively, essential oils can be used alongside breath work or other somatic exercises which may be beneficial to the vagus nerve (Mortensen, 2023).

Heaton-Shrestha (2022) also point out that there is some possibility that aromatherapy could be utilized if done so carefully within a therapeutic relationship with a psychotherapist or counsellor. She says that this could be as an adjunct to talking therapies or used as a tool during or between sessions. In Chapter 7, we will see how one aromatherapist used essential oils during coaching sessions in a drug rehabilitation centre, and another used them with clients who had been for talking therapy.

Employing essential oils to support people who have experienced trauma has many advantages. First, it is relatively accessible for most people and many of the essential oils used in small-scale studies are sustainable, easily obtainable and cheaper than pharmaceutical intervention. Second, there are fewer side effects. Essential oils are also non-addictive and easy to use. Bespoke blends can be made, and they may be used alongside other interventions such as talking therapies.

I suspect they would be better tolerated and they would facilitate more compliance than pharmaceuticals. Moreover, there is a growing demand for more 'natural' interventions and sadly a growth in people being diagnosed with PTSD (Langley-Brady *et al.*, 2023) (although, as mentioned before, I would argue that this 'figure' is not a true representation of those experiencing trauma, for the real numbers are likely to be considerably higher). We do need to see an increase in research using aromatherapy and essential oils with people who have trauma or PTSD.

Unfortunately, much of the research on essential oils and trauma is small scale and some of it is on rodents. In many instances, the methodology of the studies could be improved. Certainly, we need more human studies.

Rhind (2020) points out that there are some challenges with essential oil research. One of these pertains to the fact that because we can smell an essential oil it is hard to have a placebo control. Those being studied will be able to tell if they can smell an aroma or not, unless it is at such a low level it cannot be consciously detected. However, interestingly, there is some evidence that we may pick up low-level aromas even when we aren't consciously aware of them (Barwich, 2020; Hawkes & Doty, 2009, cited by Rhind 2020).

Scientific research tends to use a single essential oil. This makes sense as it makes it easier to isolate what works and what doesn't. It lessens the variables that could intervene and narrows down the pharmaceutical providence of the naturally occurring chemical constituents. For example, if a blend created a reaction, it would be hard to know if that was due to the entire blend or one single oil or a particular chemical component. As aromatherapists, however, we often use blends that lend themselves to creating a harmonious synergy, especially if we are working in our own clinics. There are advantages to this. For example, Langley-Brady *et al.* (2023) note that it may be most appropriate to mix a blend of four or more oils when doing reactive aromatherapy. They state this is because it is hard to pick out individual chemical constituents when inhaling a blend of oils at once, and there is less likelihood of the blend being triggering as opposed to an individual oil (Langley-Brady *et al.*, 2023). Mackereth *et al.* (2023) also concur.

We should also remember that hydrolats (also known as hydrosols), CO_2 extracts and carrier oils also have a role to play alongside essential oils. In fact, hydrolats are often preferred by aromatherapists for use around small children for safety reasons. I will discuss these in more detail in Chapter 8.

It seems that unless it is a negative trigger, aroma can be a friend when someone is living with trauma/PTSD. There is certainly a need for more research in the role aromatherapy can play, and it will be fascinating to see over time how our understanding of olfaction and trauma develops.

Finally, it is important to acknowledge that trauma doesn't have to be a life sentence. Post-traumatic growth and resiliency are possible, as we will see later, and aromatherapy can be a useful part of someone's world during their healing journey and beyond.

Reflection points

- Have you previously considered how aroma and smell intersect?
- Have you used essential oils yourself and with others?
- What are the benefits of using aromatherapy with people who have experienced trauma?

CHAPTER 6

Working in a trauma-informed way as a holistic practitioner

Trauma informed care acknowledges that many people have experienced potentially traumatic events and that the health consequences of such events are significant.

Ranjbar *et al.*, 2020, p.9

Trauma-informed care (also known as working in a trauma-informed way) is a relatively new concept in many professions. It has been driven by the health and social care and voluntary sectors but is applicable to all public services and beyond. It works on the premise that trauma is something we should all be aware of, and that we can all take responsibility to recognize and respond to it, and resist retraumatizing people when they use services.

Many of its tenets will feel familiar to anyone who has worked in counselling, psychotherapy and other settings where there is the desire to make the person using the service feel safe, and where supporting mental health and personal growth is a priority.

It assumes a position of compassion and mindfulness for the individual, with an understanding that trauma is a societal issue that can be perpetuated within structures such as healthcare (Ranjbar *et al.*, 2020). By providing trauma-informed care, services can improve conditions that can enhance healing from trauma (Fallout & Harris, 2008).

There is no definitive answer for or agreement on how to provide trauma-informed services, which is challenging when writing about it. Yet, it seems to be largely discussed within the context of what is commonly known as the four Rs of trauma: Realizing the extent of trauma,

Recognizing the signs of trauma, Responding to trauma and Resisting retraumatization. (The four Rs originate from The Substance Abuse and Mental Health Administration (SAMHSA), according to Grossman *et al.*, 2021).

By understanding the pervasiveness and complexities of trauma, and taking care not to retraumatize through our actions, words and policies, we can better support our clients. If we recognize the signs we can respond appropriately. Reading this book may be your first step in this direction, or one step of many in acknowledging and understanding these four Rs.

With an understanding of the four Rs we can then assess whether our work encompasses the pillars of trauma-informed services (safety, choice, collaboration, trustworthiness, empowerment and cultural consideration). This is where we really get to analyse our offerings to our clients.

My hope is that you will reflect on your own practice, experiences and possibilities for the future. This is not an easy task. It is not a tick-box exercise to do once and then say you've done it. This is a springboard to get started and it is something we should be continually reassessing. It is a constant process of reviewing and reflecting, considering what we offer and how we offer it. We may not always get it right, but we can make every effort to ensure that we do the very best we can, learn from any mistakes we make and improve things going forwards.

I want to also acknowledge, you may have your own experiences of trauma, and services that have responded poorly (or well) to you. If memories, feelings and bodily sensations are stirred and activated by reading this, give yourself time and ask yourself what can you do to look after yourself right now.

The four Rs of trauma
Realizing the extent of trauma
It is hoped that by the time you reach this chapter you will understand the extent and prevalence of trauma. We know we should not limit our understanding of it to only those clients who have a PTSD diagnosis or those who discuss something traumatic with us, nor can we stereotype or assume who will or won't have experienced trauma.

If you have an existing client base, can you think of clients who have disclosed things which suggest a history of trauma, or have you had clients who have not used the word trauma but have told you about events that were traumatic? Where do you think you have seen examples of generational, cultural, racial or group trauma in your practice?

What did you note? Have you talked with other aromatherapists or professionals about trauma and their experiences of it? What learning have you committed to (other than reading this book) to expand your understanding of the scope of trauma?

We should also look at our consultation/intake forms. Do we even ask the right questions? I now ask about previous traumas or experiences that the client thinks may be useful for me to know about or that they feel may have influenced their well-being.

When I spoke to naturopath Sue Adlam (who is also trained as an aromatherapist) she told me she asks her clients about adverse childhood experiences. I asked her if she felt aromatherapists needed to adapt their consultations and she said yes. She made an interesting point that while we should be interested in early adverse experiences and trauma, we should also be looking for signs of how the gut is behaving, knowing that there is a strong relationship between gut health and trauma. For example, Sue feels that it would be useful for aromatherapists to use the Bristol stool chart with clients and ask how often someone passes faeces. She reminded me this can tell us a lot about people's health generally as well as their nervous system. She told me, 'If someone is in sympathetic mode, their stool is likely to be a 1 or a 7.'

Recognizing the signs of trauma

The large list of symptoms given in Chapter 4 serves to remind us of the many ways in which trauma shows up in the body and behaviours. Symptoms of PTSD and other long-term conditions that may result from trauma can be extensive and we have already addressed these in the previous chapter. Your client may or may not be aware of their symptoms and may or may not make connections with past experiences.

Speaking with your clients and observing where they are at, on the day you see them, will indicate what needs your attention. If a client is in front of you trembling, sweating and frightened because they have just been in a car crash on the way to you (this has happened to me before), that is what is showing up and that's what you attend to.

Sometimes a reaction comes out of nowhere. It is unexpected both for your client and for you. Should this happen, the key thing is to remember to stay calm and to use a soft supportive voice, reassuring words, and your body language to let them know they are safe. We can help them remain in the present and we can attempt to co-regulate with them.

Let me give you an example. One day I was working with a lady who has fibromyalgia. At the time, she was on a waiting list for a PTSD assessment. I had seen this client many times before on an ad hoc basis. I did an aromatherapy massage and followed this with some energy work that she had asked for. During this, I felt a rush of release as I worked down her arms into her hands. We had both been silent for some time. Then she started to weep. I gently placed my hand on her arm. I reminded her she was safe and calmly asked if she wanted me to carry on or stop, all the time keeping my voice soft and gentle.

She told me, 'It just needs to come out, it's good.' She cried a lot and at times her body shuddered and trembled. I had never seen this trembling and shuddering to such an extent, but it felt right to let her body go with the flow. Her heart rate rose, then started to fall and as we started to breathe together a synchronicity came about. Later when I started to really investigate polyvagal theory and read Peter Levine's work, I looked back at this experience through a slightly different lens. I understood that I had helped her co-regulate. She was allowed to experience the bodily discharge that she needed to go through with the trembling, and she was allowed to let the tears flow.

Part of our continued professional development is that we look back at our previous experiences and learn from them. When I started to learn about immobilization as a trauma response, I was reminded of another client I saw, maybe ten years ago. She spoke incredibly quietly, she was flat and depressed, her body hunched over, shoulders drooped, making little eye contact. Honestly, I struggled to make sense of why she had come to see me when she clearly didn't seem to want to be in the room with me.

I now appreciate and understand that she was immobilizing (sometimes referred to as shutting down, or freezing, although the latter tends to refer to someone who is more static). She did not feel safe, and despite talking to her gently and agreeing on a way of working together I felt that I couldn't reach her. I also suspected that she came to see me to appease her frustrated doctor. She never returned. I wondered what happened to her for some time, and I felt as if I had let her down.

I now reflect on that experience and am acutely aware that in that instance, I did not recognize her trauma, and I don't think I met her where she was at. At this point in time, and in this context, I did not understand this dorsal state. I now know better.

Over the years, I have noticed that many people I work with have autoimmune issues, digestive problems such as irritable bowel syndrome and sleep problems. A large proportion of these have experienced trauma either as children and teenagers or later in life through their work. I'm acutely aware that it is relatively recently in my career that I have made this connection. Like everyone else, I continue to learn.

Researching trauma and really understanding its impact on the mind, body and soul also means you start to see things through a slightly different lens.

Let us take the example of pain. While many studies show that there is a clear co-morbidity between chronic pain and PTSD, some research shows conflicting results about whether people are more sensitive to pain when they have experienced trauma. It is thought that this may relate to many factors, including the nature of the trauma and other trauma symptoms. For people who are dissociating, there may be numbness, and pain sensitivity may be lessened. Remember that during the trauma their body has learned that this is how it needs to be to survive, but now the danger is over, it carries on in this mode. When you feel numb it can be hard to describe how your body feels, and sometimes you feel separated or disjointed from it. Pain sensitivity may thus be reduced, and of course other symptoms may dominate. Conversely if you experience different symptoms and are hyperaroused, for example, pain sensitivity may be increased (Tesarz *et al.*, 2020).

Lykkegaard Ravn and Andersen (2020) note that the type of trauma may also be relevant, as some subgroups report more chronic pain than others. They state that chronic pain is commonly found in individuals with PTSD, yet some people have PTSD due to the incident that caused the pain. Both chronic pain and PTSD, they note, seem to aggravate each other negatively.

They demonstrate this with an example of a patient who had been involved in a car crash. She had chronic pain from her injuries and found compliance with her physiotherapist's exercises difficult as they increased her pain, and she was worn out and hypervigilant. As she was seeing a psychotherapist it soon became evident that she had PTSD and she realized that discussing the traumatic event intensified her pain. In addition to this, doing her exercises was retraumatizing her, and because she was afraid that she would reinjure herself, fear was also a prevailing factor. Her PTSD made her feel overwhelmed. The authors also noted that she started to comprehend that her resources were being split between her pain and her PTSD, so if one was bad, it would intensify the other (Lykkegaard Ravn & Andersen, 2020).

Co-morbidity of PTSD, brain injury and chronic pain has also been realized in military veterans (Stojanovic *et al.*, 2016), and where chronic pain and PTSD correlate there is also increased risk of suicidal ideation among US military veterans (Blakey *et al.*, 2018). If you are concerned your client may be suicidal, please ask them. This will either eliminate the worry, or you may save someone's life.

Responding to trauma

We always need to stay within the confines of our role, and act professionally and appropriately with compassion and care. There may be times, however, where you are caught off guard. On several occasions, I have had someone be talking normally, then suddenly they say something that catches them. It may be a memory, an experience they had forgotten, a physical reaction, or a feeling that wells up inside them, often catching them off guard too. At times, it happens when they are silent, as if a memory in the body is somehow triggered.

You might notice a change in their body – for example, the body might jerk, arch, hunch, pull away or tremble. If you are doing aromatherapy massage it might feel as if it is rippling. Their temperature and/or breathing might change, and they may sweat. They may try to explain using words or find that words are too hard. Other people may cry, sob, howl, make another noise or weep. For decades, many holistic practitioners (especially body workers) have viewed this as some kind of release, though we haven't always had a vocabulary for it.

Having worked in information and counselling settings for years and having had some basic counselling skills training, I don't feel frightened by this. However, I can understand that it could be bewildering or unsettling for someone, especially if you find emotion difficult or it feels as if it triggers something in you.

The primary aim is to help the client feel safe as soon as possible. Staying calm and acknowledging what you see by giving it words can be helpful. We also need to check out what is happening to eliminate the possibility of a serious medical crisis; for example, sweating, nausea and shortness of breath or tightness in the chest could indicate a heart attack. Once you have done this, reminding them that they are safe and talking calmly and soothingly to them is beneficial.

If they start to seem distant, or they feel their vision is impacted (for some people in crisis things visually look different, for example as if people are further or closer away, or less clear), you can ask them to focus on something in the room, such as the feeling of their body on the chair or couch, or get them to describe a picture on the wall or feel and describe the texture of a cushion they are holding.

If they can use words and choose to share something with you, acknowledging that and thanking them for sharing it with you is useful. You can then ask them how they feel after sharing this with you. You are simply checking in with them, you are not being a therapist or counsellor. Here is an example:

> Client: 'I wasn't physically hurt but it really frightened me, and I never really got over it.'

> Aromatherapist: 'That sounds very difficult. Thank you for sharing this with me.'

> Client: 'I don't know why I thought of it, it just came into my mind just now.'

> Aromatherapist: 'And how do you feel now you have shared that with me?'

Avoiding platitudes is really important. Being told that your abusive childhood has made you the amazing strong person you are today is unlikely to be of use because no one wants an abusive childhood in the first place! It can make people feel unheard and diminished.

Your role is to be an aromatherapist who shows up in a compassionate and caring way, however you want to do this, and stays within the confines of your role. This means if a client does share a memory or expand on what has happened in your session, you don't need to ask lots of questions or ask for details of their trauma. Research suggests this is not necessary (Haines, 2016) and it is also not your job or area of expertise. You don't want to make things worse by asking for details which may only serve to further retraumatize them.

Remember that someone's experience is theirs alone, so do not compare it to yours or someone else's. In such instances, it might feel scary, surprising or overwhelming, but by staying calm and in control of your own response, you can respond in a more helpful manner. We will discuss referrals later.

It is also important to find a way for you to unpack what happened at a later point. This is of uttermost importance if you are to look after yourself and is also very necessary if someone says something that is a trigger for you. At times, as human beings we manage trauma by locking it away in a box. Some of us choose to do work on understanding what is in the box, some don't. Sometimes we think we have done all the work we needed to do on something difficult or painful in our past, and then something happens, or someone says or does something that reminds us. It can feel frightening, overwhelming and seem like a curve ball coming from nowhere.

I remember one instance when someone told me about something traumatic that had happened to them just as they were leaving my home. Work colleagues who were counsellors had told me this commonly happens in therapy work. The person may want to disclose but doesn't want to delve into any detail there and then, so they say something quickly before they leave. In this instance, what the person told me was uncomfortably close to something in my past. As the information was divulged, I felt my chest freeze. It literally felt icy cold. My stomach clenched, my head went numb and fuzzy and yet my skin prickled. Noises filled my ears, my legs felt weak, and it felt hard to breathe. It was unconscious and happened so quickly. I am almost certain I managed to hide what I was feeling (I sincerely hope I did), we chatted for a few minutes and then she left. I remember shutting the front door and trying to catch my breath and then just sitting down on the floor crying. It really took me by surprise.

Being caught unawares like this was shocking. The past can seem far away at times but close by when we least expect it. I felt vulnerable and deeply ashamed. Had I given away how I felt? Looking back, I don't think this was the case. I gave myself some grace and sat quietly with an essential oil and just breathed for a while. I considered what had happened and I was able to make the distinction between 'her stuff' and 'my stuff'. I thought about what I needed to do in the here and now to start to feel okay, aware that I had two more clients to see later that day. I cleansed the room and went to be elsewhere for a while.

It was a poignant reminder that sometimes things can happen that are completely unexpected and catch us unawares, and it was also a reminder that we all have our own wounds too. We not only have to recognize the wounds of our client, but also our own. Personal growth is an ongoing journey. We are never truly done.

In the counselling and psychotherapy world it is mandatory that you not only experience therapy yourself, but that you also have supervision. In the aromatherapy world, we have no such thing. I think this is a mistake. For starters, reflective practice is something we should all be doing on a regular basis, and in addition, most aromatherapists are self-employed and lone workers. I am lucky in that I have a good network of aromatherapists and other body workers to whom I could talk confidentially if needed (without of course revealing anything confidential about the client), but not everyone has this. Having a confidential aromatherapy buddy or mentor can be extremely useful. We owe it to ourselves to better consider how we can support one another (more on this in Chapter 9).

Resisting retraumatizing

We must take care not to unwittingly retraumatize individuals, groups or communities by what we say and do. Let us look at the example of hugging. I wouldn't normally hug a client, but I know some people in life who hug everyone. Unsolicited touch for many people simply doesn't feel safe or okay and we must always respect that. We can maintain boundaries and we can follow our clients' lead.

Van der Kolk (2014) gives an illuminating example of a young woman in a mental health institution being restrained and force fed. He noted that she had been abused earlier in her life and he wondered if that experience had retraumatized her. Physical contact can easily be retraumatizing for some, so we should take care, ask permission and explain, if we are providing a touch modality such as massage or acupressure.

There are many things we can do to help our clients feel safe and not retraumatize them. I always make sure that I explain to my client other noises they may hear. Something that would be meaningless to one person is not to another. For example, hearing other people moving around elsewhere in the building, on stairs and in corridors, can be unnerving. This is especially important for people who have experienced abuse and or sexual violence. Elaine Le Feuvre tells me she also talks to her clients about the noises they may hear, and sometimes demonstrates these (e.g. by opening and shutting her cacao cupboard), so the noise sounds familiar.

Working in partnership with the client, clearly explaining things and asking permission, preserving their privacy and asking for consent are simple but effective things we can and should do to resist retraumatizing. If you need to break confidentiality or connect with another health worker or agency to keep them safe, you can involve your client in this process.

I do corporate clothed massage as well and on more than one occasion clients have disclosed something that has made me concerned for their safety. In those instances, we can talk openly with our client and remind them of the confidentiality policy we discussed when we first saw them and explain why we need to speak to someone else. In every instance of this, the person has given me permission to break confidentiality. Letting them know that you are concerned about them (or someone else) and that you have a duty of care to tell someone else helps them understand why confidentiality needs to be broken. There are sometimes ways to involve them in that process, for example they may prefer to disclose the issue to someone in human resources but have you present, or they may prefer you to create that dialogue but they don't wish to be part of it. By working with them in this process (where possible) we can avoid retraumatizing them, and encourage them to have control in the situation (something that has normally been taken away in the experience of most trauma).

On a greater scale, we should be thinking about our business policies and mission statements, or those of the provider we work for. The language we use is also important and can convey realized or unrealized prejudices. Lewis-O'Connor *et al.* (2019) remind us that health and care services can unintentionally be part of, and add to, trauma through implicit and explicit bias. This bias may occur for several reasons, such as historical trauma, intergenerational trauma or institutionalized trauma, according to Menakem (2021).

Reading Menakem (2021), I came across research he cites by Hoffman *et al.* (2016). They found that out of 222 white students a shocking 40% of first-year students and 42% of second-year students believed that black skin is thicker than white skin, and 8% of first-year students and 14% of second-year students believed that black people had less sensitive nerve endings. In a comparison with a group of 92 white lay people, 58% thought black skin was thicker and 20% thought black people had less sensitive nerve endings (Menakem, 2021).

Clearly this is factually grossly incorrect. The colour of someone's skin does not mean that they have thicker skin or less sensitive nerve endings. Yet these are chilling statistics that help us understand how racial bias can mean that people are let down by health and social care providers, and this can include complementary therapists such as aromatherapists. This bias ends up creating further trauma.

A healthcare provider who makes assumptions about the sex of someone's partner, or a receptionist who can't find an appointment for a disabled person because all the appointments with the doctors are upstairs that day, are examples of institutionalized bias, whether intentional or accidental. These are things that to an outsider may seem small and accidental, but to an individual they can be repeated time and time again, each time adding layer upon layer to existing trauma. Even the language we use is biased – think about the term dis-abled, which assumes 'abled' is the way we should be. We surely need to constantly check in with our own bias and assumptions. This can be extremely uncomfortable and difficult, but it is necessary.

Pillars/principles of working in a trauma-informed way
Safety

There are so many aspects to feeling safe during a session with an aromatherapist or other complementary therapist. This starts from the very first time you communicate with each other, whether this is by email, telephone or online booking. You may work somewhere where appointments are made for you, and your first experience will be in person, or you may offer virtual appointments online. You may speak to the person directly before you book them in.

Safety can refer to many things including (but not exclusively) knowing what to expect, confidentiality, consent, the consultation process and feeling safe in the physical space you work in. It can also relate to privacy and boundaries. I will expand on some of these below. I have chosen to expand on the topic of safety, because it is so essential in relation to trauma.

To feel safe myself, I very rarely work with anyone unless I have spoken to them, or I know the person who has referred them. This gives them a chance to ask questions and helps me gauge a little about their situation and why they want to come and see me. (It has also been very useful in identifying the occasional person who states they want a massage but really they want something else inappropriate and illegal! Unfortunately, those of us who offer aromatherapy massage sometimes get implicit or explicit requests for sex or sexual acts.) It also offers the client a feeling of safety.

Before we meet in person, I help set the scene. I check that they know I will send an email with the address and directions. I describe the building and the drive, so they know where to park. I explain that there is gravel outside, and two steps into the building and that my treatment room is downstairs, next to the door with a toilet nearby. There are things our clients should know beforehand. For example, if you are working from home and you have a dog, you need to tell your clients that. What if they have been bitten by a dog and are frightened of them, or have allergies? I also describe other possible noises they may hear, such as loud bangs if there is building work nearby.

Everyone has the right to privacy. For those of us who work as aromatherapists and offer body work alongside this such as massage, explaining the process is essential. Clients should know how to get on the couch, when they will undress (and how much), how to use the drapes to cover themselves and that you will knock before entering. We can explain how we use the drapes.

I have been for body work before where the therapist thinks simply turning their back on me is enough for my privacy. It doesn't feel professional or safe for most people, because the therapist has all the control – they can turn around at any minute or see you naked in the reflection of a screen/piece of high gloss furniture/mirror.

Privacy also relates to the information clients share with us, and often overlaps with confidentiality. In the UK, we need to make people aware of how long we legally need to keep their records for, their right to see their information and who they can complain to if they think their data is not being stored correctly.

To my mind, an aromatherapist shouldn't be telling other people who is or isn't their client (though I have met several complementary therapists who think it is okay to do this). Our clients can share that information with whomever they want, but it isn't our job to do so. When I do my first consultation with my clients, I address what I offer and how I work, and I want to find out why they are coming to see me and what their goal is. Before I go through my consultation forms, I need to address confidentiality and spell out very clearly what that means. If you work in a clinic, hospital setting or other social/healthcare setting you are likely to need to follow the confidentiality policy of the institution you work for. If you are going into such a setting as a self-employed person, you need to have that transparent conversation with the service provider, so you can be clear with your clients.

Discussing confidentiality is paramount to safety both for your client and others. If someone is about to reveal something, you can remind them of your policy, thus giving them a choice. Should you have to break confidentiality it is important to state why, remind them of your policy and your previous discussions and try to work together, as this is more empowering.

Consultations also need to feel safe. This can be encouraged by explaining why you are asking the questions you are asking and what you will do with that information. You may wish to use scales such as the Body Perception Questionnaire[1] to assess the autonomic nervous system, in which case explain a little about these to your client and gain permission. New Zealand aromatherapist Annie Price (2021) asks clients during their consultation to circle words that describe their predominant feelings over the last few months. She asks them not to analyse them, noting they could add their own. The words are a range of positive and negative emotions.

In some instances, clients may have a session booked for them which they haven't consented to. This can happen in a multitude of ways. Someone who is ill, infirm or no longer has their faculties may not be able to consent to treatment. This does not necessarily mean we do not treat them. I gave an example earlier of taking aromatherapy into a special needs school. One young woman did not like touch and therefore there was no way that would be incorporated into her aromatherapy. She could not verbalize this with words, but her body language (such as turning or pulling away, lack of eye contact) and noises she made suggested that she did not want touch for whatever reason; her key workers were aware of this, and so aromatherapy was not offered through that medium. People's ability to feel safe needs to be respected.

Consent may also be called into question if a person has a progressive illness and cannot verbally consent. However, in many instances they may have previously enjoyed a hand or foot massage, so their treatments might continue. In such instances, we watch all the while for clues from them as to whether it still feels safe or wanted. And what of working with people when there is a language barrier? How do we ask for consent in these situations? There is much to consider.

On occasion, people are given vouchers for services as a gift. Most of the time these are non-returnable, but what if someone doesn't feel safe coming to see you (for whatever reason)? Are there other services or adjustments you can offer instead? Someone who is agoraphobic after a trauma may not want to leave their home and come and see you. Could you offer a 'virtual' appointment and then follow up with a personalized product sent to them at home instead?

Physical privacy is also integral to feeling safe and this can be offered by drawing blinds, using screens, robes, drapes, leaving the room if someone needs to undress, and knocking before returning. Many people feel shame and embarrassment about their bodies and therefore it

---

1   www.traumascience.org/body-perception-questionnaire

isn't appropriate to make comments about someone's body that do not pertain to why they are with you.

Many years ago, I went on an advanced massage course. Now, as body workers when it is our turn to receive the treatments, we are normally happy to leap on the couch at lightning speed, as we are so pleased to receive the work ourselves. I did just this, and the lady who was practising her work on me made a comment on my body size (something along the lines of 'there is barely anything of you') as she draped me. I was very slim at the time and had had numerous comments about being skinny over the years (including several assumptions as well). Comments in the past were often unkind but, in this instance, the comment really didn't bother me at all, and I did not think anything of it.

The body worker teaching us called her out on it immediately, telling her in no uncertain terms that she should never comment on a person's body size. The lady practising on me was mortified and nearly in tears (I recall I ended up reassuring her). I took nothing negative from the lady's comment at all, nor was I offended. While the teacher was not helpful in the way he managed it (he loudly told her off, shaming her in front of the entire class), he was probably right to address it. The way in which he did this could have been better though. As I write this, I see how ironic it was – he told her off for body shaming and then shamed her, and who knows what this brought up for her.

What seems like a seemingly innocent comment to one person is not to another. A friend reminded me of this in a group discussion many years ago. Another mutual friend was talking about food and what she should and shouldn't eat. My friend quietly and calmly said that people should let her eat what she wanted to eat, because it is not helpful to try to control other people's food intake when they have a history of an eating disorder. No more was said on the matter. Ripples of trauma can lie behind many 'everyday' conversations.

When I worked with counselling and information services there were several things that would be included in the room set up to protect the client and ensure as safe a space as possible. One of these was for them to be able to see the door and to sit nearest to the door. When we chatted about her work, Cynthia Tamlyn also reminded me that many people with lived experience of abuse do not like to have their back to a door.

Good lighting outside the building, and soft lighting and comfortable furnishings inside a room also help a space feel safe (the latter being more challenging after COVID-19 when these had to be removed and everything was being constantly wiped down). In public buildings like hospitals there may be bright strip lighting and sometimes this can be turned off and lamps used instead.

Some people work with music and others don't. I do both, depending on what my client prefers. I have a white noise box which plays alpha music and clients seem to love this. Some people find silence uncomfortable. On the odd occasion when I have not had access to music (for a technical reason), people who don't like silence have preferred to chat. Clients should be given the choice where possible.

There is a school of thought among complementary therapists that you should not let your client chat away. I firmly believe that it is their time and their choice. If they prefer doing this, that is fine with me. The difficulty is (especially if you are a chatty person like me), knowing when to stop or slow this down. Sometimes trauma (or even just life generally) can make people feel very lonely, and comfortable chatting can help us feel more socially connected and engaged (as we saw in polyvagal theory).

Traumatic experiences can often socially isolate people, and in such instances, we become part of someone's support and resource. I had a lady who came to see me some years ago as her normal aromatherapist was currently unable to work after an operation. She was a carer for a terminally ill partner and she wasn't able to get out much. In fact, her aromatherapy massage was her only respite. One day, she came for an aromatherapy massage, and towards the end she told me that her previous aromatherapist was now returning to work and that she wanted to go back to seeing her. I had assumed this would happen and I said I was happy to hear that her normal aromatherapist had recovered, that I had enjoyed working with her and I wished her well. 'She knows everything about me, and it is like putting on a comfy slipper', she said. It was what she knew, it felt like the best fit, and, importantly for her, it felt safe.

Maintaining our boundaries is important for both our clients and our own safety. Janina Fisher (2023) explains attachment trauma can lead some people to become over-clingy and over-invested in relationships and this has implications for people working with them.

This is interesting when I think of my experience as an aromatherapist. Many of us have had clients with trauma histories who struggle with change. I recall once telling a client that I would be having two weeks' annual leave soon and that her next appointment would need to be in three weeks' time. She looked at me in panic and said, 'But what will I do? I don't know if I can wait that long.'

This was quite challenging because obviously an aromatherapist is as entitled as anyone else to take holiday, and, momentarily, I felt as if there was an expectation for me to change my holiday plans. I pushed this thought aside and we talked about things she could do for herself between appointments, such as self-massage with a blend. I made a blend for her that she was familiar with from previous sessions. I wanted her to reach a place where she could manage the gap without needing something from me, and that did happen. We want to encourage our clients to come to a place where they feel able to have the resource to manage and are not over-reliant on us.

What I realized later was that my client was saying, 'I am not okay with this, my body/mind/spirit needs the support.' Perhaps she struggled because it activated her sense of being abandoned.

This realization came in very useful and now if there are bigger than normal gaps between appointments (e.g. over Christmas), a handful of clients who might find this gap more difficult to manage choose to have their favourite aromatherapy blend in a bottle of carrier oil (so it is diluted at the same ratio as when we use it in the treatment room). They can either self-massage, ask a loved one to massage them or I suggest smelling it, or rubbing it on their hands, arms, feet and chest (especially across the CV17 acupressure point), and sitting and doing some breath work or meditation. This is empowering and avoids over-reliance.

Choice

How can we offer our clients choices and involve them in their aromatherapy experience without overwhelming them? We can ask simple questions, such as would they like us to adjust or change the lighting, temperature or sounds in a room? We can assess if they have any aroma triggers or negative associations with aromas, and check their smell preferences.

We also need to be mindful of not predetermining the aroma before people come to see us. For example, it has become quite popular for yoga teachers to use a diffuser in class, but have they assessed if anyone has aroma triggers, allergies or sensitivities? When offering several aromatherapy appointments in a day, it is important to air your room as much as possible to allow aromas to linger less.

Giving people choice allows them to be part of the process and not feel 'done to'. This is important because many people who are particularly marginalized and traumatized may already have less choice. Someone living in temporary accommodation, a refugee centre, domestic violence refuge, rehabilitation unit or prison will have less choice over many things most people take for granted, such as their daily activities, who they can socialize with and where (if at all), the food they eat, the clothes they wear, if they can go outside.

Dina Nayeri (2020) writes about the shame and guilt of refugees continually being expected to feel grateful, even though they have so few choices in life. Some people will also have historical trauma (e.g. genocide or medicalized trauma) of being 'done too' or having their rights taken away, so choice and empowerment become even more important.

I'm extremely mindful when doing body work of asking before touching, and giving the client choices. Let us imagine I think it is a good idea to put a bolster under someone's knees. I can tell them that by adding a bolster under the back of their knees they will probably feel more comfortable. They can agree or disagree. If I point this out, people will normally lift their knees ready for me to do so. If they want the bolster but don't do this I can ask, 'Could you please lift your knees so I can place the bolster under them or if you prefer, I can lift your legs and slide it under. Which would you rather do?' The point is that the choice is theirs, and I don't suddenly touch their feet when they don't expect it because they have come for a back, neck and shoulder aromatherapy massage.

People who have medical conditions or have had surgery have sometimes experienced medicalized trauma, and it is crucial that as someone who is trying to support their health, we do not perpetuate this in any way. Similarly, survivors of abuse, violence and human trafficking have had things done to them against their will. The likelihood is that you may never know this. Given that Rape Crisis (2023a) suggest one in four women and one in eighteen men have been raped or sexually assaulted in their lifetime as an adult, we should be working with the assumption that a proportion of our clients have had this experience. In some communities and client groups these figures may be even higher.

Collaboration

When we work with someone, we work side by side. We recognize the other person's input and we do not 'do to'. We collaborate and agree on a way forwards in how we will work together. We continue to explain anything new and ask permission along the way if we think deviating from the plan is a better way of achieving their goal. While we work with essential oils and our knowledge, they are showing up and working with themselves. Of course, our essential oils, hydrolats, CO_2 extracts and carrier oils are also doing the work.

There are many aspects to collaboration, including checking out smell preferences and choosing blends or checking on pressure if incorporating aromatherapy in massage, asking them for more information where needed, exploring options together, coming to agreements and obtaining permission. Collaboration needs to be a partnership as you work towards your agreed goal.

Good collaboration allows us to make the most of our strengths, skills, resources, knowledge and experience, and encourages us to thrive. Collaboration can also be empowering as it levels up the balance of power, because we don't want our clients to be passive recipients. Collaboration happens on an individual basis but can also happen at a wider service delivery level.

Many service providers collaborate with clients on how they provide their services, what they can do to eliminate barriers to access and ways in which services can be improved. Collaborating in this way can help develop services that best meet the client's needs. A term you may come across when considering how you collaborate and empower clients is co-production. For more information on this, visit the Social Care Institute for Excellence.[2]

Information can be gathered in multiple ways. Most commonly this is verbal feedback or feedback exercises in person (on a one-to-one or group basis), written, online or telephone questionnaires (with the option for these to be anonymous), or focus groups (in person or virtual). Each way of gathering information has its own advantages and disadvantages.

True collaboration with service users/clients within the health and social care sector can make a massive difference in tackling barriers of inequality that by themselves can be part of structural trauma.

Obtaining feedback on services is more common in health and social care, but as lone workers with our own businesses, we can also find ways to collaborate with clients on the services we provide. Even simply sitting side by side with someone and filling out the intake forms rather than asking a set of questions could feel more collaborative.

Trustworthiness

Trauma (especially complex trauma) can mean that making and maintaining relationships is particularly hard and this can impact the client and aromatherapist relationship. So, what can we do to build trust in

2   www.scie.org.uk/co-production/what-how

our relationship with our clients? It helps if we can be open and honest about expectations. An example of this can be exploring boundaries such as telling your clients what hours you work and let them know that if they contact you outside these hours, they are unlikely to get a response until you are next back at work.

A project offering complementary therapies to victims/survivors of trauma in the southwest of Northern Ireland consulted its service users. Out of the 150 consulted, trust in their therapist was highlighted as an important aspect, with the report stating it was something that the participants were vocal about. Professionalism, approachability, experience, and a personal grounded approach were all seen as building towards feelings of trust. One participant said that after 30–40 years of 'being suspicious' it was hard to stop being suspicious, but trust was built through the therapists helping people feel at ease, being calm, not rushing people, and being seen as friendly and experienced. One comment was, 'They are trustworthy and confidential – you felt you could tell them things' (South East Fermanagh Foundation, 2012).

Empowerment

Validating people's experience, feelings and reactions can be a powerful way of letting people know that you have heard them and are being empathic. Many people who come to an aromatherapist may spend more time talking to us than anyone else about their health and well-being. Denise Cusack told me she had worked with some war veterans once a month for an hour, over four years. One told her that he had spent more time in consultations with her than he had with medical personnel in his entire life. The power of a listening ear, within the context of our work, should never be underestimated.

Supporting clients to take control (e.g. self-referring when they find this possible) may be useful. The very nature of our work means we can support them in feeling more empowered in understanding how their body and mind work and connect.

There may be times where we need to break confidentiality, for example if someone reveals they are self-harming. Involving them in that process (if they wish), as already discussed, can be empowering. Empowerment can also come through your client being reminded of the steps that they have taken to change things in their lives and meet their goal. As we work with clients, we often see many changes brought about by the work they are doing with themselves. Acknowledging this is important.

Even the questions we ask on our intake/consultation forms can empower people to disclose something traumatic if they feel it is relevant to their health or wish to tell you. Lewis-O'Connor *et al.* (2019) recommend asking a broad question such as, 'Have you any life experiences that you feel have impacted your health and well-being?'

Someone I see regularly recently disclosed something from her childhood, telling me she had not spoken about it to anyone. She felt shaky and tearful, so afterwards we spent time helping her feel calm and grounded (which is often the primary goal of our session). I find Cedarwood atlas (*Cedrus Atlantica*) to be one of the best essential oils for this. Recognizing resilience is also deemed to be useful, but we have to explore what we really mean by this.

Encouraging or acknowledging resilience is different from unhelpful platitudes that may leave people feeling unheard (such as 'wow you are so strong'). For example, someone told me a while ago that her childhood had been neglectful. She had learned to fend for herself from an early age and had to look after several siblings. She had very strong feelings about her childhood and how she wanted something different for her children. 'I need to break the cycle', she told me. I let her know that I could tell from all the things I knew about her and her family that she clearly had well and truly broken the cycle. We can remind someone of their resilience and strengths without adding clichés.

Cultural consideration
To be a culturally responsive trauma-informed service, it is necessary to appreciate and understand that culture influences much of our life, including our traditions, belief system, goals and expectations, existential concepts, communities and relationships. As such it can also affect how people interpret and respond to trauma (National Institute for Health and Care Excellence, 2018). Additionally, it can influence whether people seek support in the first instance, who they seek it from and the way in which services are accessed.

While Elliot *et al.* (2005) remind us that it isn't necessary to know everything about every culture, it is important to recognize that different cultures may vary in how they view things, including the meaning of certain traumas, support systems, resources and healing.

Ranjbar *et al.* (2020) give an example of an Indigenous American teenage boy Pepe. After a series of earlier traumas and more recent aggressive events (including his own suicidal thoughts), he was taken to an inpatient psychiatric unit where he was diagnosed with a psychotic disorder and given medication. When returning home to his community his experience was described differently to him by a local spiritual healer. Pepe was, the healer said, experiencing a spiritual crisis. Yet with ceremonial and community support he could become a traditional healer, like his great grandfather. His trauma was interpreted, understood and treated in a different way from the approach his psychiatrists had. Crucially, the authors noted, it also offered a resource for healing.

Ranjbar *et al.* (2020) suggest that physicians approach their work with cultural humility, noting that in our work with others, we also need to be aware of our own cultural backgrounds and our implicit bias. I think this is wonderful advice for anyone working with others.

Culture may be one of many barriers to accessing services, but there are many others, including (but not exclusively) economic class, sex and identity, religion, age, disability, sexuality, race, refugee status, homelessness and educational background.

Work on your own wounds

Psychotherapist Carl Jung coined the term 'wounded healer'. He understood that many people come into healing professions with the desire to help others, and that this is borne from their own wounds (traumas). When I mentioned on social media that I was writing this book, several aromatherapists contacted me to say that their own experience of trauma had led them to want to do holistic 'healing' work with others.

Being a wounded healer has benefits, such as potential increased empathy and, in some instances, understanding how to navigate a medical, social care or other system (because the healer has been through this themselves). Wounded healers can also bring hope and resilience to their work (Newcomb *et al.*, 2015).

There is of course a potential risk of transferring their unmet needs onto the client, and inappropriate self-disclosures can occur. Newcomb *et al.* (2015) also found that there is an increased risk of secondary trauma. I believe all student aromatherapists should be taught listening skills and be made aware of the risk of secondary trauma. They should also understand that they need to be willing to work with their own wounds too, through talking therapies, somatic work or other forms of exploration. Aromatherapists can also try to understand how to manage any situations in which they might find themselves triggered. During our discussion about trauma, Donna Robbins told me how she thinks about triggers: 'When we are triggered, it is just our bodies trying to keep us safe. I have learned that a trigger is a fabulous learning opportunity and that this is a possibility for me to become more empowered in myself.'

Florian Birkmayer is a well-known figure in the aromatherapy community, with a background in psychiatry and addiction work. He says aromatherapists, 'need to embrace their own wounded healers' journeys to stop unconsciously asking their clients to carry their woundedness in a shadow projection and stay trapped in the client role' (Birkmayer, 2022, p.37).

The difficulty is that with many aromatherapists working solo, there are few, if any, support provisions in place, unless that aromatherapist has made great efforts to create their own. In other professions this is normally offered. When such topics are neglected or brushed past in initial training, within continued professional development and within governing bodies, we can lose these essential concepts that keep our clients and ourselves safe and our relationship healthy.

One way to combat this is to join a regional network of aromatherapists or have a buddying/mentoring system with a peer with whom you have a trusting relationship. Anything confidential that would give away the identity of the client of course cannot be disclosed, but it does provide the opportunity to reflect, develop new skills and share any difficult or challenging moments. Clinical aromatherapist Emma Charlton (2023) suggests that the keys to successful mentoring include making a confidentiality agreement, dividing the session equally for both of you, reminding yourselves of the principles of active listening, presenting alternative ways of doing things in a constructive manner and agreeing on frequency. The sessions should be taken seriously, like any important meeting should.

Seeking a trauma-informed aromatherapist or other professional

If you are reading this with a view to finding an aromatherapist (or any holistic practitioner or body worker) who is trauma informed, there may be a few questions you may wish to ask before booking an appointment. I always welcome a conversation first and no longer book anyone in unless I speak to them first.

Here are some typical questions that I have been asked:

- 'What makes your service trauma informed?'

- 'What is your experience of working with someone who has trauma?'
- 'I have had xyz experience when having a previous aromatherapy massage, so I am keen to have one again but without this experience. Can you offer this?'
- 'Why do you think aromatherapists need to be trauma informed?'
- 'Does trauma really show up in your treatment room?'

Post-traumatic growth

You may have heard the term post-traumatic growth. The concept refers to the idea that personal growth and transformation can come from surviving trauma. It brings a sense of hope, meaning that trauma does not have to be a life sentence.

Tedeschi and Calhoun (2004) remind us that it does *not* mean that trauma is good or desirable, nor does it mean that personal growth only comes from trauma. They comment that we must understand that growth occurs in the context of distress and suffering. For many, growth will co-exist with distress from the trauma, and we should be aware that not everyone finds post-traumatic growth.

They also note it is crucial to realize it is not appropriate to talk about post-traumatic growth with people until they have done plenty of work on healing their trauma wounds. Telling someone that their trauma has made them stronger, as we saw earlier, is an unhelpful, patronizing and trite platitude because the trauma and the impact of it isn't positive, nor is it an experience that people would wish to have (Tedeschi & Calhoun, 2004).

As we have already seen, personal experiences may drive someone into a career that they then flourish in, where they can support others or, as Herman (2023) says, they may find meaning in their trauma and realize it is part of a wider societal problem, which can lead to campaigning for change. For example, in 2020, Sarah Super managed to campaign for a memorial to survivors of sexual violence in a park in Minneapolis (Herman, 2023).

Artist Andy Farr (who created some amazing paintings based on several people's lived experience of PTSD) commented in an interview about his work, that he had not appreciated the impact of post-traumatic growth for people at the beginning of his project. One of the people Andy painted told him that after he had healed from his trauma, he became more musically creative (Woods & Farr, 2019).

Menakem (2021) reminds us that trauma may inhibit our ability to learn, grow and change, but tells us that once it has been addressed there is the capacity for growth again. Our brains are remarkable, and plasticity continues throughout our life.

As I was exploring the idea of post-traumatic growth, I remembered the work of Lois Tonkin on grief from courses I had co-written. Led by her work with bereaved clients, Tonkin postulated that we don't 'get over' or 'move on' from the grief of a loved one. Instead, we grow our world around it. Rather than grief reducing or going away, life starts to develop and expand. The grief is still there, but life around it grows so it takes up less metaphorical space in the person's world (Cruse, n.d.).

This seems a wonderfully applicable model for us to think about with post-traumatic growth. The trauma doesn't 'go away', it is still there, and there are likely to still be triggers and distress, but it doesn't control or constantly impede our physiology, minds or behaviour.

Reflection points

- If you work as an aromatherapist or in another role within an organization, what can you do to ensure that your practice is more trauma informed?
- What are you doing to work on your own wounds?
- How can you avoid vicarious/secondary/indirect trauma?

CHAPTER 7

Using aromatherapy when trauma is present – case studies

The discipline of aromatic therapy has allowed us to reconnect aroma with healing.

Rhind, 2020, p.39

As aromatherapists, we are in a unique position to be able to support our clients.

American Aromatherapist Jade Shutes summed this up brilliantly in a session she ran on trauma and resilience for an international conference, when she said that aromatherapists can create anchors, safe spaces, rituals and tools for people to widen their window of tolerance (window of tolerance is a term coined by Dan Siegel and it describes the optimal 'window' or zone in which someone can manage their emotions) (National Institute for the Clinical Application of Behavioural Medicine, n.d.).

Our aromatic tools can help our clients feel grounded and secure. Furthermore, an awareness of their process of smell, plus any additional exercises (e.g. breathing exercises) or associated modalities, such as massage or self-massage, can help them feel present in their bodies. By working together with a trauma-informed aromatherapist, they can feel supported. We can offer a safe space, a holistic and thorough consultation, and a compassionate and professional approach.

I wanted this book to shine a light on the valuable work that many aromatherapists are doing around the globe, using our aromatic substances with clients who have experienced trauma. These are just some examples…

Working with babies and children –
foetal and developmental trauma

Some aromatherapists (who have the correct training) will work with pregnant mothers, children and even babies. In these instances, the range of essential oils or hydrolats used, the amount used and dilution rates are radically different. Some essential oils should be avoided for safety reasons.

We should always bear in mind that the foetus, babies and children are still developing, so if you are not trained in this field, please seek the advice of a qualified aromatherapist before embarking on this route.

It is essential that, where possible, children have some sense of partnership when working with an aromatherapist. American clinical aromatherapist Cynthia Tamlyn tells me that giving her client control is paramount, whatever their age. This also extends to giving them the choice of whether they use the aromatic product or not. Cynthia specializes in working with adopted children, and both children and adults who have experienced paediatric trauma. She only uses hydrolats with children under the age of five years old. When I interviewed her, I discovered that she likes to really find out about the child's world, asking them questions such as what their favourite colour is or who are their favourite TV characters.

Cynthia gave me an example of a little girl she was working with who had only slept through the night three times in four years. Together they created a custom-made blend of hydrolats and called it her 'freedom to dream' blend. This was kept in the fridge and when she started to feel that everything was getting too much, she could run to the fridge, close her eyes and spritz her blend, allowing the tension to melt.

Using her blend, the little girl was able to start to sleep through the night, which was one of the goals they had been working towards. Interestingly, Cynthia told me that although her clients may start with aromatherapy, once the initial goal has been met, they often then move onto another complementary modality. In essence, the aromatherapy has done its work, allowing them to move in another direction. In the example she gave, the little girl was then supported by equine therapy, once she got to a point where she finally felt comfortable leaving the house.

My former career in counselling and information services for children and young people taught me that working sensitively in collaboration with a child or young person is important in any therapeutic relationship. It allows choice in a world where they have often had few (if any) choices available to them. For a child who has experienced abuse, or for one who has a medical condition requiring surgeries, medications or procedures, choice around their body has often been taken away from them. It is therefore crucial not to perpetuate this, however well-meaning.

Aromatic therapy can become available even at a pre-verbal age. American clinical aromatherapist Lora Cantele told me about an experience she recalled many years ago, when she provided aromatherapy for a distressed baby. The baby's mother was a crack addict and the baby had been born with some level of brain damage, the extent of which was unknown. The baby was inconsolable and continuously crying. The nurses in the children's home where she lived would desperately try to calm her. Lora said:

> I made baby products with Sweet orange (*Citrus sinensis*) and Lavender (*Lavandula angusitfolia*) essential oil (bath wash and lotion). I also made a blend that was diffused in her room. It helped to comfort and console her. It helped her stay calmer and sleep. The problem was when there was a shift change and the baby was passed from one nurse to another, she would start crying all over again. To help this, I put the diluted blend in a spray and had the new nurse spritz the front of her smock before accepting the baby. The baby then identified the scent with comfort, thus accepting the new person caring for her. Her mother rarely came to visit, but when she did the baby rejected her and would be inconsolable. We started using the spray on the mother and it helped the baby to accept her holding her and put a nervous mother at ease.

Working with drug and alcohol addiction

Saboohi Khan is a clinical aromatherapist working in Pakistan. While working as a student aromatherapist, she conducted three aromatherapy case studies at a male substance abuse recovery rehabilitation centre, over a four-and-a-half-month period. Saboohi worked closely with the centre's experienced clinical psychologist and had her school principal for support and mentoring.

Working within a residential drug rehabilitation centre came with certain constraints, meaning Saboohi had to think creatively about how she could apply her skills. For example, she could only use aromatherapy in a way that would impact the individual (and not other residents), so using a diffuser was not possible. She was also not allowed to use anything in a bottle (as this could look like or be reminiscent of a drug), so instead she decided to use personal aroma inhaler sticks, asking participants to pick a colour that they were most attracted to. All three picked yellow – this choice of a bright sunshine colour was perhaps related to the lack of garden or outdoor space, Saboohi thought.

Saboohi is also trained as a personal coach, so she incorporated some of this experience in her sessions alongside the aromatherapy.

Due to the risk of the inhaler sticks going missing, being stolen or being used by someone they were not intended for, the men were not able to keep their inhaler stick. However, they could access them for two or three minutes via the clinical psychologist who saw them daily, or other ward staff. Initially, they were used three times per day (morning, afternoon and evening), but this was then changed to two times per day in the third month as they wanted to reduce any sense of reliance on it.

When Saboohi had the first and second session with each client, the clinical psychologist at the centre was present for the first ten minutes. This helped to establish rapport and create safety, trust and familiarity for everyone. Saboohi told me she wanted to work in a non-judgemental and open way, with the goal being 'to get them to fall in love with themselves and to feel they are worthy of the life they have'.

Over the next four-and-a-half months, the men had 10–12 sessions, that were 45–60 minutes long. Saboohi would start the sessions by asking her client what they would like to cover that day, what would add value to their week and what emotion would they like to focus on. The aroma inhaler sticks were often used alongside breathing techniques or progressive muscular relaxation techniques.

Being set up this way, the session had a focus with a mutually agreed outcome. She explained that this also meant that clients created a strong emotional anchor to the essential oil.

After each session, Saboohi would meet with the clinical psychologist, so they could assess how the client was doing. The clients were aware of this interaction, and Saboohi describes the work as a real team effort.

Two clients were immediately attracted to an essential oil, but one client had very limited olfaction due to his drug use. He could only smell Peppermint (*Mentha x piperita*), Lavender (*Lavandula angustifolia*) and Spearmint (*Mentha spicata*). Saboohi opted to use Spearmint with him, because she was aware that he had used Vicks vapour rub while inhaling drugs, and Peppermint seemed far too close in aroma, and Spearmint is gentler.

By the third week, Saboohi noticed that the essential oil inhalers were becoming a 'supportive friend', helping her clients start to get in touch with their feelings. This was impactful as they were used to a cycle of shame and feeling alone. Around weeks seven to eight she noticed a shift happening, as her clients were asking more questions rather than the other way round. They were also able to express their emotions more freely. One client told her, 'I know now what it really means to care.'

Saboohi gave me an example of using Petitgrain (*Citrus x aurantium*) with one client. The aroma would remind him of times collecting harvests and sitting under a tree in a field. Working with the inhaler stick, he was able to have more difficult conversations about the violence and anger in his past that had led to him losing his job and becoming violent towards his wife. He was able to begin to talk about his son. This client responded well to blends with Rose (*Rosa damascena*), Ylang ylang (*Cananga odorata*), Bergamot (*Citrus bergamia/Citrus aurantium ssp. bergamia*) and Petitgrain.

Looking objectively at these choices, I found his essential oil preferences intriguing. All these essential oils typically lift the mood and imbue a sense of happiness: Rose would nurture his soul and promote self-love, Ylang ylang would bring confidence, Bergamot and Petitgrain would diffuse anger and frustration. It is as if he knew exactly what he needed – perhaps unconsciously he did.

The project showed some key positive effects for the men. It helped them access and explore their feelings and consider and work with obstacles in their life and it brought positivity into their daily routine. One client said it helped his moods, remarking, 'I feel better and more at peace, by working on my behaviour via this therapy.'

Another explained that he used to feel hopeless and anxious. He commented, 'This therapy was quite beneficial...the use of the inhaler kept my environment and day quite smooth and reminded me of the things I had discussed with my coach.'

Saboohi also noticed that one client she had taught box breathing to then went on to teach this to other residents.

As Saboohi talked about her case studies, I was impressed with not only how hard she tried to help them have useful tools, but also how she was able to think creatively about how she could best support her clients. Saboohi saw benefits to both her clients and her, stating that her work was 'a mutually healing journey'. She poignantly reflected on her experience, saying, 'Essential oils can bridge the silent communication gap and create a soul-healing experience, loosening up the verbal communication channels, to feel safe enough to express the patients' emotional needs.'

One case study that was particularly fascinating was one man who had been at the centre for almost a year and had been very limited in his participation. With aromatherapy treatment and coaching, things seemed to change.

In 2023, I attended a continued professional development (CPD) talk by clinical aromatherapist Victoria Plum at the International Federation of Professional Aromatherapists' annual general meeting. The talk was on working with clients who are substance addicted and one of the things I was particularly struck by was how she noted that essential oils would help her clients feel safe. She said that she had felt that many of the clients she saw came into the world feeling unsafe.

Victoria also mentioned how many were taking a lot of medication and/or had complex medical histories, so she preferred to work with a smaller number of oils and would use ones that had no contraindications, such as the restricted essential oils we might use in pregnancy. She worked at low dilutions (1% maximum, or even less).

She also found that her clients were often hypersensitive to the subtle energies of the essential oils. I have also found that clients who are particularly aware of their trauma and trying to work through it can be more sensitive to touch, pain, movement and, interestingly, essential oils. During her talk, Victoria also suggested that we should ask ourselves, as aromatherapists, if our presence felt safe for them – and, if we are using a touch modality, if our touch felt safe for them.

Observing and checking in more regularly with your client is often necessary when they have a history of trauma. Checking in with ourselves is also needed. Victoria told me after her talk, 'I believe we, as practitioners, really need to be grounded, supremely calm and spacious so that we model the sense of safety to help the client find that in themselves.'

Working with clients after a natural or accidental disaster

In June 2017, London saw a tragedy unfold as a tower block caught fire claiming at least 72 lives. Clinical aromatherapist Jane Lawson went down to the site with a colleague within days to see if complementary therapies could be offered to the surviving residents and the fire crews. Jane described it as 'like walking through a war zone. People were literally "leaking", tears running down their faces.'

It was clear that complementary therapies such as aromatherapy could be offered, but she and her colleague decided that whoever wished to join the therapists had to be vetted first, with their insurance and professional training certificates checked.

Jane told me that it was such a shocking sight she decided that everyone who wanted to work as a therapist there needed to go and visit the tower block first. This was useful because some complementary therapists realized that the sight of it was too much, and they were not emotionally equipped to volunteer. Jane felt that this was a valuable exercise because what she saw in real life bore no resemblance to what was being shown on TV.

Jane noted that people were initially in survival mode (or what is known as reactive depression). The complementary therapists ended up working in a few different places across the next few months, with the final residence being a large warehouse locally. The sessions they offered were free of charge, and clients had two to three therapists assigned to them, covering their different health needs (both as a result of, and prior to, the fire), such as acupuncture, aromatherapy, massage, reflexology, kinesiology and energy therapies. Each person had a lead therapist, which was useful for collating information and progress. Some of the therapists had previous experience of working in communities traumatized by war.

Initially, clients had two to three sessions per week. Jane revealed that the initial focus was to ground them by addressing their reactive depression. I asked her what difference the sessions made for clients, and she replied, 'People reacted very quickly and positively to the combination of therapies we prescribed for them individually, and as a result, they were able to get on with life.'

One client who particularly stood out for Jane was a young man we will call John. John had lost his family to the fire. Shortly after the fire, a colleague asked Jane if she would see John. He was loud, twitching and agitated, swearing and noisy and the NHS psychology team were threatening to section him. Jane described how John was yelling and was unable to stand still. She grabbed bottles of Vetiver (*Chrysopogon zizanioides*) and Fragonia (*Taxandria fragrans*) essential oil and took him outside.

Jane invited him to talk to her, and while he was talking noisily and angrily, she wafted the Vetiver close to him, while holding a stress point on his knees, a technique she drew from kinesiology. At one point he asked, 'What is that, it stinks?' She told him it didn't matter what it was, he just needed to keep talking. He did and after a while gave a big sigh. Jane knew the Vetiver had done its work, as he had stopped swearing and shouting, so she switched to Fragonia, wafting it under his nose. He calmed down further and then gave another big sigh before starting to cry. After a while, he thanked Jane and said no one had just listened to him before.

After six months, the therapists were asked to leave, and the project ended. I asked Jane if, after her experience at Grenfell, she had any advice for other aromatherapists looking to set something similar up in the future. She felt that there were a few things she would advise, including vetting therapists really well so they were experienced, making sure they saw the site of the disaster so they fully understood what had happened for their clients, having good communication between therapists, setting up measures to ensure that people do not abuse the system (e.g. pretend they were a resident when they weren't), writing it all up afterwards and collating it. The latter can be useful for many purposes, for example if there is an enquiry, or to inform peers about disaster relief work.

Jane also mentioned that people would commonly forget things about their health and because of the shock, they weren't always able to think straight. This illustrates how important it is to use essential oils that don't have lots of contraindications. A smaller group of essential oils, with limited or no contraindications, may be needed in disaster relief work, partly because it isn't practical to carry lots around, and also because it is hard for people to remember their medical history in such circumstances.

In late August 2005, the USA experienced hurricane Katrina. The hurricane was to spawn 62 tornados in eight states and caused approximately 80% of New Orleans to be flooded within 24 hours. An estimated 1200 people lost their lives, and it became the USA's most expensive hurricane, costing 108 billion US dollars (Britannica 2023a).

Three years later, clinical aromatherapist Fusako Takada went to the area. There was still a massive displacement of people, with the impact still being keenly felt. Many residents were not aware they lived in a flood risk area and had no insurance. With waters reaching up to 8 meters, many people had lost everything. The flooding happened at the end of the month when people on low incomes were already struggling, and recovery had been tremendously difficult. Of her experience, Fusako said:

There were many individuals still living in trailers even three years after the storm. I visited those people, one trailer at a time, with a local pastor. I had a massage oil with Lavender (*Lavandula angustifolia*) in my bag and I gave hand massages to people every time I met someone. The scent of Lavender comforted the person, got them relaxed and they became talkative, often talking about their experiences.

Many of the people she saw were the elderly, who were not able to start again somewhere else (or did not want to as they had lived in New Orleans all their life). In many cases, their children and grandchildren had moved to other cities to start afresh. Fusako said, 'The scent of Lavender made people more talkative. Another good thing was that I wasn't from New Orleans, and that made me easier to talk to.'

Perhaps the Lavender opened people up, allowing them to talk of what they had seen, smelt, heard, felt and experienced. As Fusako noted, she was an outsider, and perhaps this gave the people she saw permission to freely tell her their experiences. After all, she had not been there before, so she had no attachment or loss connected to the area. She told me:

Many people mentioned their insomnia, muscle pain (stiffness in the back and shoulders) and loneliness from being away from family. They observed many people passed away around them...suffering from heart attacks and cancers as time went by, and many experienced depression and suicide.

Fusako went to a church service one day and afterwards was approached by a young man who said he was thankful for the massage she gave his mum. Fusako had found the lady being chatty and friendly, but the young man told her that she had struggled with depression and been feeling quite down. After her aromatherapy hand massage, he said she had felt so much better.

In March 2011, Japan experienced a terrible tsunami and earthquake which is estimated to have killed between 18,500 and 20,000 people (Britannica, 2023b). More than half of these were aged 65 and over. It left widespread damage and created a nuclear emergency. Fusako travelled to some of the villages affected the following year.

Fusako's friend had previously stayed in a trailer and provided aromatherapy support to people affected. She made a sleep balm and a muscle balm as people were troubled by insomnia and cramps or stiff neck and shoulders. Fusako said it was very difficult for people to be in temporary

accommodation throughout the winter, as it is very cold in Northeast
Japan at that time of year. Her friend led classes to create balms, and
these were welcomed by the local government as they became a way
for people to socialize and meet new people. So, when Fusako went
to Japan her friend shared these recipes and Fusako was able to create
some balms in advance to distribute to everyone in temporary housing.
She also gave hand massages where she could. One of her friends also
started to have nightmares, due to hearing so many people's traumatic
experiences (which suggests secondary trauma). Fusako told me more
about her experiences working in traumatized communities:

> I blended Lavender (*Lavandula angustifolia*) and Grapefruit (*Citrus par-
> adisi*) essential oil into massage oil and gave massages to people who
> were staying in temporary housing. Most of these people were elderly.
> They loved their hand massages, although some of them were hesitant
> to receive it initially because people in the Japanese countryside are shy
> and not open. In Kamaishi, my friend was leading craft classes. One day
> she took me to one of the apartment complexes that was rebuilt after
> the tsunami and earthquake. I won't forget that experience. Though
> we were there to support those ladies, they were preparing cakes and
> pickles for us. They suffered a lot but still shared what they had with
> others. Their kind gesture really touched my heart. When I massaged
> their hands, I was really surprised, because those ladies had hands that
> were bigger and thicker than other women's. They enjoyed their hand
> massages, and some of them shared that they had lost their husbands.
> The area was called Kirikiri and was close to the area called Otsuchi
> where the entire city was swept away by the tsunami. The tsunami was
> huge, so it just uprooted and washed away the whole city. That was
> such a tragedy.
>
> There was one lady who was hesitant to receive a hand massage in
> the group. She eventually came to me and said, 'You know until today,
> there were many volunteers who came to us. Some did hand massages
> like you are doing, and I never let anyone do it to me, but I let you
> massage me today because I like you a lot.'
>
> She seemed a bit nervous when I started to massage her hand but
> then relaxed by the end. She was hurt by being regarded as someone
> who needed help. The tsunami and earthquake forced them to be in
> that position and for some it hurt their pride. They were strong and
> independent people in the fishing industry, then the disaster suddenly

left them helpless. Until I met that lady, I did not realize that some people in the countryside are shy and not so open.

We also visited another temporary housing place on our way from Kirikiri. I met another lady who had lost her husband in this tsunami. She was so calm, smiling and gentle. Losing her husband must have been a shocking event but she calmly said, 'I am thankful because there are people like you who are coming over to care for us.'

In Ishinomaki, I met a lady who failed to escape when the tsunami came but managed to stay on the second floor of her house with her husband. They only had a couple of bottles of water. This was all they had until the water was gone. They were totally unprepared. While they waited for the waters to recede, they saw people they knew drowning before their very eyes, but they were not able to do anything because the waters were too powerful. After the water was gone, she struggled with her emptiness and once wished to die because she wanted to escape from the trauma.

My friend eventually moved to the city, but she shared with me that she started to get insomnia after hearing many stories like this. Although she did not go through the actual tsunami, she started to experience the shock that those individuals went through by hearing their stories, and she started having nightmares about tsunamis.

Disaster experiences are so shocking and unique because if you break up with your spouse you still have a house and a job and so on. If you lose your job, you still have family and a place to live. Disaster can take everything from your life in a second, with no choice. You cannot prepare yourself for this. It often leaves people in strong shock.

Working in a country that has seen multiple traumas

Nicole Boukhalil is a clinical aromatherapist working in Lebanon and she told me, 'In Lebanon, we are undergoing a continuous state of trauma...the trauma is affecting everyone.'

The country experienced decades of war (which Nicole said no one talks about), and in 2019 the country experienced a massive crash in their currency which led to most people financially struggling. Pensions and savings became redundant. Then in 2020, COVID-19 happened. This came at a time when hospitals were already at breaking point, with staff not being paid and shortages of medical supplies. This was then followed by a huge explosion in a port in Beirut which caused over 200 deaths and thousands of injuries. An estimated 300,000 people were made homeless. The blast was even heard in Cyprus, more than 150 miles away. Unfortunately, the country was already experiencing crisis in accessing medications due to massive shortages. Uncovering exactly what happened in the blast has been difficult. Nicole told me, 'We were just supposed to go on and live.'

Talking to Nicole, I realized just how complex things are. She sees continuous examples of trauma among her clients, with panic attacks, insomnia, depression and other mood disorders being common. She said she sees a lot of depression in older clients particularly. Not only have they lost their financial security, but they have a deep sense of losing their country, their roots and their homeland. Many are losing their families too, as younger family members move to other countries to seek out a different life (which Fusako also noticed was happening in New Orleans and Japan).

Being as simplistic as possible in her offerings is one of the keys to Nicole's work. She told me that the simple things are the things that bring help and security. For example, in Lebanese homes, it is commonplace to find Rose (*Rosa damascena*) or Neroli (*Citrus x aurantium*) hydrolats, and they are often used in cooking. As such, they are very familiar smells that often evoke memories, as the country grows many bitter orange trees and roses. She often uses a mix of these two hydrolats for people to spray around themselves when they feel the need, and clients tell her they find it comforting.

While Nicole, as an accomplished aromatherapist, is clearly aware of the emotional properties of these hydrolats, her rationale for using them is also based on this cultural familiarity. Cedarwood (*Cedrus atlantica*) is an especially important essential oil, as Cedar is the national emblem of Lebanon. She told me that almost everyone would be familiar with the tree and said, 'In our unconscious, we know that this is a tree for solidarity and strength.'

For aromatherapists, Cedarwood has an amazing ability to ground and root us.

She also finds she uses a lot of Angelica root (*Angelica archangelica*) and Fir essential oils, the latter being particularly useful for allowing people to breathe more openly. She also uses Bay laurel (*Laurus nobilis*) (which again is commonly used in food), finding it useful for confidence and the respiratory system and noting that it seems to help people 'do things and go further'.

Nicole explained that many people find they have difficulty breathing and that they often feel trapped.

Nicole also uses blends of essential oils in aroma inhalers as she finds these can be easily used by people. Keeping things simple is important when people are traumatized because brain fog and memory issues can make complicated things more challenging.

We talked about the process of smell and how trauma can impact it and Nicole told me about a time she made something up for a client, and although he was involved in the whole process and said he liked the blend, he never used it. Remembering this she said, 'It was as if he didn't feel anything...or didn't want to feel anything. Maybe he wasn't allowing himself to smell, to remember, or to open up.'

As she spoke, I was humbled and reminded of the importance of understanding the cultural resonance of aroma, and the nuances of the trauma. The experience of trauma may be very specific to a country, culture or region and can have many intricate layers.

Working with refugees

Natascha Köhler is a paediatric nurse and aromatherapist who has been volunteering in refugee aid since 2015, working, for example, in refugee camps in Turkey. She says that essential oils are useful for protecting her against colds in stressful times and are hugely helpful for refugees. In an article she was interviewed for, Natascha describes how much children loved the cheerful smell of Lemon (*Citrus limonum*) essential oil and how she would make roses out of paper napkins and sprinkle them with Lemon essential oil. When she went home, she left behind jars impregnated with Lemon essential oil so they could constantly return to the smell of Lemon (Golla, 2017).

> I worked with refugees in camps in Turkey and Greece. In my backpack, I had several essential oils, some Almond oil and little empty bottles. In seconds, there were a lot of people, everyone had problems, and everyone needed help. It was loud and there was not much space, but when I opened essential oils and they started smelling the different essences it became quieter. Everyone wanted to smell and so I had the opportunity to look at which essences the person in front of me liked. Their reaction to the different smells was a good lead for mixtures. I mixed lots of recipes, with hundreds of eyes following what I was doing.
>
> I tried to give them good experiences with smells they would know from their home. A lot of the refugees I met were from Syria and Afghanistan and they were used to Rosewater. When I opened the bottle, the

women started smiling, and led me to understand that they used it for cooking as well as perfume.

They were so far away from home and had fled from a terrible war. They were not welcome no matter which country they arrived in, and they had no idea how the future would be or if they would be able to go back to their roots. I always had the feeling that the smell of rose aroused memories in a good way. It was familiarity, an anchor.

When I prepared for my first trip, I had lots of diseases in my mind and so I mixed a lot of oils for the skin and coughs but when I was in the camps, I realized the trauma that they were suffering. I hadn't had to experience what they saw in war or on their flight to the refugee camp, but in the camps, I saw their circumstances, and the effect on the soul, and so I mixed the trauma oil.

Natascha kindly shared her recipe with us.

TRAUMA OIL

10ml Sweet almond (*Prunus amygdalus dulcis*) carrier oil
1 drop of Spikenard (*Nardostachys jatamansi*) essential oil
1 drop of Cistus (*Cistus ladaniferus*) essential oil
1 drop of Rose (*Rosa damascena*) essential oil (pre-diluted at 10%)
5 drops of Neroli (*Citrus x aurantium*) essential oil (pre-diluted at 10%)

Natascha told me:

> The work is the most satisfying work I have ever done but you also have to look after your mental health. I left after two weeks but a lot of locals stayed and helped every day, so I mixed oils for them to save/ protect themselves.

She kindly shared the blend she left behind for her colleagues.

SAVING OIL

30ml Sweet almond (*Prunus amygdalus dulcis*) carrier oil
2 drops of Cistus (*Cistus ladaniferus*) essential oil

5 drops of Lavender (*Lavandula angustifolia*) essential oil
5 drops of Neroli (*Citrus x aurantium*) essential oil (pre-diluted at 10%)
5 drops of Rose geranium (*Pelargonium x asperum*) essential oil
3 drops Rose (*Rosa damascena*) essential oil (pre-diluted at 10%)
10 drops of Lemon (*Citrus limonum*)

Natascha reflected, 'This work is only a drop in the ocean, but one drop of Lemon for the children gives a thousand smiles.'

Denise Cusack is an American clinical aromatherapist who has worked with Herbalists Without Borders (HWB) for years, responding to fire, flood, hurricane, street protests, war, refugees, veterans and more. She explained beautifully in her own words how aromatherapy can be a powerful tool in such environments:

Aromatherapy products are easy to explain or demonstrate, even with any language barrier or no previous aromatherapy experience. They are portable and easy to distribute. When working with folks who have experienced trauma, cultural relevance can make a big impact – meaning using aromas from the culture of the people using aromatherapy.

While there can be physically negative responses to aroma (smoke after forest fires, for example), and there is also a big impact of using an aroma from home and family when people have relocated to new places, especially under stressful and traumatic situations.

When working with Afghan women, we discussed using Rose (*Rosa damascena*) essential oil in combination for inhalers and an infused lotion for sleep and calm. Therapeutically, Rose is used during times of emotional and physical stress, soothing and calming both the body and the mind. For the refugees, it is an aroma of home and comfort, traditions and even food. It is calming and luxurious and supports healing and making a person feel cared for. While it can be expensive, Rose is also very strong, and even a drop in a chest rub or lotion, or in a blend that is dropped onto inhalers, can be optimized to get benefit without great cost. The aroma of home and comfort, combined with the therapeutics of working with essential oils, makes a big impact.

While we always hear back when people love a blend that has been made and distributed in our work, we also can see the visceral response and body language as people open and smell something for the first time, reinforcing that we have made a good choice.

When we go into relief work, care kits work well in that we can also label things in multiple languages in advance, knowing who we are serving. So, working along the border of Mexico in the US, we know that labelling in Spanish is a priority. Preparing items in advance helps with good labelling – and in relief we usually know the main types of needs we will see, such as trauma, stress/anxiety, sleep and skin issues, and any needs related to the season and location. If we make those items in advance, we are preparing everything in a sanitary space, labelling it with multiple languages if needed, and sorting things by need or creating care kits that can be passed out. When working in a clinic environment, making things in advance is also helpful, as we are often working outdoors, in tents, in refugee camps, and do not have the ability to custom blend for every individual. With clinics, however, we can do an abbreviated intake to hear the primary needs and concerns, and then choose from our pre-made selection of items to dispense to the person. Having handouts pre-made with instructions is helpful as well.

Relief work can meet those immediate and critical needs, but it can also be educational. Many refugee situations have people living for long periods of time in camps or in shelters, and people get bored and are stressed in an unfamiliar environment. Hosting free classes to teach people how to make their own inhaler or rollerball can be a way to engage and get to know people better. People feel that they are doing something to help themselves and their families.

In education, speaking the language is very important, so that we are empowering people through education, and not imposing over them. For a rollerball class, take a set of five blends in a bunch of dropper bottles labelled clearly in the language spoken by the group. Take carrier oil (bottled down into many smaller bottles). Take funnels, empty roller-balls and either pre-printed rollerball labels (for the five blends) or make pretty blanks that people can draw on, so provide waterproof, fine-tip, colour markers. Have some instructions in the language of choice that are out on the table for people to read. If other indigenous languages might be present, have someone come to translate.

Share about the plants, the oils, the benefits and the uses, and let people pick their own. This can be relaxing, fun, enjoyable and educational, and it is also an activity that can support people dealing with stress and trauma.

When choosing how to use essential oils, it can depend on the supplies, environment, time, language, and location, in addition to need. When serving first responders who are battling forest fires, you will know that the needs might be not only stress, but also stinging eyes, respiratory and sinus inflammation, chest congestion, and difficulty sleeping. So, when you make first responder care kits, you might look at making chamomile eye tea bags, an 'open air' inhaler, a 'breathe easy' chest rub or lotion, a calming bedtime pillow spray, and a tea blend for a wet cough. If you will be there passing them out, you can talk people through it, share how to use them, and what to do. If, however, you are setting out a care station for anyone at the shelter, you will need clear instructions on the products and/or a handout in multiple languages, if possible, with very clear instructions.

I personally love creating blends that address not only trauma, stress and anxiety (which is present in all work of this kind), but also the feeling of self-care, and that someone is caring about them by giving them something lovely. Including aromas that are culturally important, something they feel perhaps that they would never get because they are not worthy, makes an impact on many levels. Aromatherapy can do all those things. Thinking of the people as individuals and how they have been impacted and might feel as they enter our environment and creating something that will make them feel special and cared for is important.

One year, a member donated many bottles of St John's Wort (*Hypericum perforatum*) oil to the network for clinics along the US border in Tijuana. Every single bottle was carefully wrapped in lovely ribbons stitched around a gauze fabric that had 'You are loved' stamped in Spanish. It made me cry, and I heard back from people distributing them that it made people cry to receive them. While that may seem as if it takes time, energy or money, it really was more about the care and saying that people are worthy and deserving. This can make an impact alongside the amazing aromatherapy and herbal tools we have.

The importance of reminding people that they are loved and worthy of care is something we see throughout this chapter. Denise told me that in general relief work, where people are living in tents, it is best to avoid cold-pressed citrus essential oils due to the phototoxicity. She said:

I prefer to always blend items at a lower concentration into rollerballs, lotions, rubs or inhalers, rather than giving people straight essential oil blends unsupervised. Always assume that even if you tell people not to put it on their children, that they might, so prepare gentle and safe blends (which are still amazing and effective).

Ancestral trauma

Cathy Skipper and Florian Birkmayer specialize in working with ancestral trauma, to help people stop unconsciously replicating the traumas of previous generations. Cathy outlines the major stages of this in one of her many informative blogs on her website. She talks of confronting the trauma using a grounding essential oil, then using another oil such as Labdanum for understanding the trauma, and moving on to feel and release the historical trauma (for which she suggests Everlasting), and finally connecting with and beholding the ancestral clan, for which she suggests Marigold essential oil (Skipper, 2020a).

Together Cathy and Florian use different forms of plant medicine, working in quite a unique way. Cathy explained, 'Fundamentally, we hold space for the client, and we use aromas to facilitate their process' (Skipper, 2020b).

I find Cathy and Florian's work intriguing, and I should point out that much of the work they do is specialist and supported by Florian's background in psychiatry.

Cathy mentioned that unlike the conventional medical system they can give their clients much more time, a comment that was echoed by many of the aromatherapists I spoke with. Aromatherapists often have the added benefit of more time with clients, but how we approach the mind and body connection is different in our community from much of modern medicine.

In modern medicine, we still often see a disconnect, a separation if you will, of the mind and body and the experiences people have in their lives. Indeed, Porges critisizes this Cartesian dualistic thinking that the mind and body are separate (Porges, 2022).

Trauma specialist Gabor Maté constantly reminds us of this failure to unite the mind and body. In *The Myth of Normal* (Maté & Maté, 2023), he tells us that when he gives talks, he asks the audience who is under a medical specialist (in his words a medical 'ologist' of any sort, e.g. a cardiologist). He then asks out of all those hundreds of people who have their hands up how many have been asked about their life histories, trauma and past experiences by the specialist. He said just a few hands remain up (Maté, 2019). Time to be interested in clients' experiences, lives and goals is one of the privileges we have, as aromatherapists. Addressing all aspects of the person, and not splitting the mind and body up is, in many aromatherapists' minds, essential.

Working over Zoom with war veterans

Denise Cusack worked with a veterans' resiliency holistic clinic for several years. Through Zoom sessions, Denise would look at herbs, supplements and aromatherapy use. Denise noticed differences between male and female responses to aromatherapy:

> With veterans we did have women, but we also had many men who were not interested in diffusers or chest rubs. For them, finding ways to utilize aromatherapy that could fit into their lives but also felt right for their tough persona was important. Education might include more about the science and the chemistry of aromatherapy, rather than the emotions. Also, a foot bath or shower fizzy would be used every time, but a pillow spray before bed, not so much. A foot ointment or beard oil would be used, but a rollerball would not.
>
> Many disabled veterans did not have bathtubs or could not get in and out of baths, but they all had a turkey pan or bucket. Putting in an essential oil blend that was mixed with Dead Sea salt, carrier oil and Epsom salt enabled them to experience the benefits of not only an Epsom soak, but also the aroma from the hot pan. For many, this was the first time they had done something to take care of themselves. They enjoyed that their often-painful feet and ankles would feel better (as would their mood). They would feel relaxed and calm before bed. Drinking a steaming cup of tea while soaking in a calming and pain-supporting foot soak could be very impactful.
>
> Muscle and joint rubs/ointments were wonderful as well, and several even had their own personal formulas that would be made and shipped to them monthly based on their needs. Having significant pain from war injuries as well as PTSD and stress meant we could combine blends with that in mind and support them in many ways.
>
> Women veterans often loved having the inhalers and sprays, as they spent many years working to be more tough and less feminine, and many experienced not only physical ailments but physical traumas as women. The calming stress support and lovely aromas would work so well together.

Working with the trauma of serious illness, critical or terminal care

In clinical settings, aromatherapy is increasingly embedded into the care of very frail patients. Madeleine Kerkhof, a clinical aromatherapist in the

Netherlands, gives some beautiful examples of using CO_2 extracts (in which she is an expert), essential oils and other aromatics in her book *Clinical Aromacare* (2023).

She mentions one instance where she was asked to attend a man in his forties who was in a coma in the intensive care unit after complications from heart surgery. His wife was desperate for him to recover enough for a very necessary heart transplant. With her, Madeleine assessed his situation to see if there would be any safe oils that might trigger his senses and bring more comfort. His wife mentioned that pizza was his favourite food.

Madeleine decided to use Sweet marjoram (*Origanum marjorana*) CO_2 extract, resonating with the scent of oregano, often used in condiments. Sweet marjoram CO_2 extract is 'high in sabinyl hydrate acetate, which is responsible for that typical scent'. This would be a safe extract, resonating with comforting memories.

The scent was notably calming for him, and his wife who was also traumatized by their ordeal. Madeleine blended it with some carrier oil for his wife to use for gentle massage, which reconnected them in his final few weeks.

Jonathan Benavides is a clinical aromatherapist and psychologist working primarily in the Netherlands. In 2023, I attended a talk he gave on working with women who survived breast cancer (Benavides, 2023). He told the audience, 'Cancer is an inevitable trauma for patients.'

He observed that the trauma began with a diagnosis and that fear would be a reoccurring emotion throughout their cancer journey. Jonathan described working in a beautiful, integrative way with his clients, starting with where they are at, with the goal of alleviating some of the PTSD symptoms they experience. He uses techniques such as relaxation exercises, self-guided imagery, making a 'new me' perfume from essential oils, and teaching them how to self-massage. He poignantly noted, 'When they massage their scars on the outside, they are really massaging their scars on the inside.'

As breast cancer is one of the more common cancers, most aromatherapists will have experience of working on someone who has it or has had it at some point in their career. I remember working with a lady in her forties quite early on in my aromatherapy career. She had previously had breast cancer resulting in lumpectomy surgery. A year down the line, she had many issues with her shoulder, which was why she initially came to me. As we worked on her shoulder she would often talk about her diagnosis and the treatment she had received. This would not be the first or last time that I realized that as I worked on area of the body, a person would start to discuss what has happened to them and how it has affected them. For many, it seems it can help them process the enormity of what has passed or is happening and find some inner peace. Colette Sommers gives a beautiful example of this in my previous book (Nagle-Smith, 2024) where she saw a woman for several sessions following her breast cancer treatment.

People with serious illness, long-term medical conditions, disabilities or injuries often have so many hurdles to overcome. There may be negative side effects of treatment, physical changes to the body (and the emotional adjustment to this), unpleasant and invasive treatment or surgery, inability to do things they could previously do due to fatigue and other symptoms of the illness, restricted mobility (and potentially freedom, e.g. to leave the house, travel long distances), financial hardship, loss of career, and even a need to move home into more suitable housing. Freedom to manage personal care may be impacted. Relationships and sex life may suffer or break down. People's physical ability to care for their children or other family members may be reduced and their social life can be affected, which can lead to isolation. This can have an impact on the entire family.

In end-of-life care, the patient's family are also suffering. Denise Cusack told me that she once designed an aromatherapy garden with a hospice. She explained:

> While those going into hospice can use aromatherapy support in their final days, the people who really needed support were the family members visiting their loved ones – perhaps for the final time. In sketching out plant ideas for their garden such as lavender, rose, peony, dianthus, stock and other aromatic plants, we also talked about making a blend that smelled of the garden for people to take with them in an inhaler or rollerball. That idea was a big hit, and fresh flowers could go into the rooms, while the rollerballs were appreciated by family (and used on their loved ones).

The trauma of grief

Many trauma professionals now recognize that grief can sometimes be traumatizing. Unfortunately, those who surround someone impacted in this way do not always understand or appreciate this. I have lost count of the number of times I have heard clients say, 'Everyone thinks I should be okay' or, 'They expected me to cope and I had to do everything' or, 'I've been asked if I am over it. I will never be over it.'

Clients whose partners have died (especially when it is early, in their forties or fifties) will tell me they feel cheated of the future and that their experience is minimized by others who expect their grief to be over within six months to a year. Others will tell them they know how they feel and then compare it to losing a parent or grandparent, and later moan about their husband or wife in front of them. People with children are also trying to manage their own grief and support their children.

The bereavement charity Cruse (2023) states that while traumatic bereavement may come about from suicide, violence, accidents, terrorism or drugs and alcohol, it may also result from any sudden or unexpected death, or where someone has borne witness to the suffering and pain of a loved one. I would argue we have to be mindful of how a bereavement leaves someone feeling, rather than just look at the event.

When I met Rea, her husband had died three weeks earlier. A family member had been seeing me for aromatherapy massage and had asked if she could make an appointment for her mum. I agreed, but said it was essential that her mum only come if her mum wanted to come and see me. This was ethical as it gave her mum the choice.

When Rea arrived for her appointment, she was extremely polite. I explained how I worked and what I offered and asked if she would like to go ahead. She said she would, and we talked about the consultation form and what the focus of her treatment should be. She said she didn't really know what she wanted, she just felt awful and didn't know what to do with herself. She wasn't eating or sleeping well. She wept a lot, and we took our time filling out the consultation form. She continued to carry on and would regularly say, 'I'm sorry, I know there is nothing you can do, I know you are not a grief counsellor.' I let her know that although I wasn't, this time was for her, and it didn't matter if she cried, talked, didn't talk, expressed emotion and so on. It was a safe space for her to just be.

Rea decided she would like a back, neck and shoulder massage, perhaps with some work on the face and head. My intention was to work calmly and slowly, to help soothe her soul, and calm her breathing, as she was taking lots of double breaths after each episode of crying. In my experience, when people cry a lot, experience severe stress or anxiety or are in shock, they often don't breathe very well. This can continue and may later get diagnosed as hyperventilation (over-breathing) syndrome.

Rea told me she really liked floral smells, and I noticed the moment I met her that she wore a strong, heady, floral perfume.

I created a blend of Rose (*Rosa damascena*), Ylang ylang (*Cananga odorata*) and Cedarwood (*Cedrus atlantica*), and Rea liked it. She had had several massages in the past and normally associated them with spa days she had enjoyed. I find it useful when people are breathing poorly to try and breathe slowly and deeply when I work. They then tend to mirror this and as such we are encouraging co-regulation which is helpful from a polyvagal point of view. In those days, we did not have this concept to work with, we just knew that people would become calmer, and their heart rate would reduce. I continued to see Rea for about three years. During this time, grandchildren were born and life started to become more bearable. In time, I saw less and less of her. Many years later I saw her while I was out one day. She was well, chatty and vibrant and told me all her news. Rea didn't need her aromatherapy massages anymore, but she said they had given her some peace at the worst time of her life.

Private practice settings
Scar trauma and accidents
Clients sometimes feel very disconnected from their body when they have experienced trauma. UK clinical aromatherapist Donna Robbins spoke to me about the physical and psychological benefits of scar tissue release work with clients. She explained to me that such focused work often helps clients come to terms with parts of their bodies they feel dissociated from, especially areas that they associate with trauma. She explained, 'When I do scar tissue release work, I try to encourage my client to describe their relationship with their scar.'

She does this by asking them to grade their scar physically and psychologically on a scale of 1 to 10.

Donna gave me an example of a lady who had undergone breast reduction surgery. Her client had felt pressured to have the breast enlargement by a previous toxic partner. She decided to have the implants removed as she felt they were interfering with her health and well-being. After the surgery, she was left with big anchor scars. Donna told me that her client was disassociated from her breasts. She couldn't feel parts of them, nor did she want to. She felt angry. Her new partner was nervous to touch her breasts and they no longer gave her sexual pleasure. Over the sessions, her relationship with her breasts started to change. The circulation in the area increased. Donna finds such feelings are also common with caesarean section scars, which in some instances are a physical reminder of birth trauma.

She finds that scar tissue release work transforms the connection to the body, and helps people reintegrate parts of themselves they find difficult. As we were talking about the impact of trauma Donna told me that she believes 'trauma shatters the psyche'.

Many years ago, when Donna was teaching me to massage on my aromatherapy diploma, I remember her telling us a story about how the body stores memories of trauma. She gave the example of working on someone who was her case study when she was learning to massage. She knew the person quite well and had already given him several massages. Her client had been working outdoors in a dream job he adored. One day he was involved in an accident using a chain saw. He had surgery immediately and luckily managed to keep his arm.

Her client had a previous history of childhood trauma and seemed quite broken by the hiatus in his career caused by the accident. One day, Donna was giving him an aromatherapy massage. While working on his arm she felt the energy shift, and she described this to me as a thick syrupy atmosphere. She did not understand what was happening, but she stayed grounded and focused on the highest good. Suddenly, he sat bolt upright taking a sharp, noisy intake of breath and she described another shift in the energy that was 'like a glitch in the matrix'. Her client was very emotional and there was a real sense of shock for him and a feeling of vulnerability.

When he felt able to talk, her client explained that he saw a flash of white light, that it was very like an Indigenous cleansing ceremony he had experienced shortly after his accident.

Donna did not carry on massaging the arm but did stay holding it while he talked. We talked about how he had felt safe enough to be emotional and vulnerable, and Donna commented, 'It is an honour, that safe space that we can create.'

Violence
UK clinical aromatherapist Caren Benstead told me about her experience working with a young woman who had been attacked. Months later she came for a consultation. Caren explained:

> While her body had taken a few weeks to heal, it seems the emotional healing would come a few months later. Being alone was terrifying but

being in the outside world was worse. She had found a counsellor whom she had connected with, and as well as wanting to ease some tension in her body, she wondered if I could create a blend to support her in her counselling sessions. As her mind was busy with racing thoughts of danger, loss, grief, depression and crippling anxiety, we created a personal inhaler that was simple to use, efficient in its delivery and easy for someone with a burdened mind.

We focused on using the inhaler when she felt safest (at home), for a period of three weeks, and then started to introduce the aroma in situations where she felt uneasy and to lean on the aromatic association we had now established as a place of ease and safety. I offered my client some essential oils, but her body rejected many until we arrived at our blend.

Caren and her client created a blend of 2 drops of Frankincense (*Boswellia carteri*), 3 drops of Petitgrain (*Citrus x aurantium*), 1 drop of Palo santo (*Bursera graveolens*), 2 drops of Grapefruit (*Citrus paradisi*). Three of these essential oils had significance in terms of pleasant smell memories for the client. 'Frankincense drew her mind back to moments in church, a place of safety and peace with her family; Petitgrain from sweet holiday memories; Grapefruit from her uplifting and refreshing breakfasts.'

Caren, using her intuition, then suggested Palo santo. The intention, she informed me, was for the blend to bring comfort (from previous happy memories), peace and rest.

Aromatherapy to rebalance after a therapy session

Elaine Le Feuvre is a clinical aromatherapist. Elaine specializes in women's health and has had several referrals from local psychologists/counsellors. She found that when clients came to see her after talking therapy they were sometimes shaking and distressed by reliving their experience.

Elaine was seeing a lady who was perimenopausal. She had been involved in a traumatic incident and was now having counselling. She would come to see Elaine after her counselling sessions, with her aim being to use aromatherapy to rebalance her nervous system, increase her self-care and find ways to self-soothe when needed, as she was having panic attacks. In the short term, Elaine was also trying to help her understand the energy of each essential oil and how this interacted with her body.

She came to see Elaine for a weekly 60-minute aromatic reiki session, for four weeks. Elaine also made her a bath soak to be used for a 20-minute bath before bed, and an inhaler for immediate use when needed.

For the inhaler, Elaine used 6 drops of Nagarmotha (*Cyperus scariosus*) for its grounding and rooting subtle energies.

Her client's bath soak was aimed at soothing her nervous system, helping with irritable bowel syndrome and promoting a good night's sleep (her sleep was being disrupted by perimenopausal issues). The soak included 250g of a mix of salts (Dead Sea salt, Epsom salts, and pink Himalayan salt), a blend of 25 drops of high altitude Lavender (*Lavandula angustifolia*), 10 drops of Roman chamomile (*Chamaemelum nobile*) and 40 drops of Sweet orange (*Citrus sinensis*). She chose Lavender for its soothing, sedative capabilities, Roman chamomile for its sedative and deeply calming impact, and Sweet orange for its sweet aroma and digestive qualities, as her client's irritable bowel syndrome was made worse by stress and poor sleep.

For the weekly aromatic reiki sessions Elaine would start with breathing exercises. She explained how she arrived at her choice of essential oils in the first aromatic reiki session, where she used one essential oil for each chakra:

> I chose high altitude Lavender for the crown chakra (associated with spirituality) over regular Lavender as its higher linalool content is more anxiolytic, calming and soothing, helping to ease the overthinking mind, and reduce stress.
>
> Blue lotus (*Nymphaea caerulea*) (for the third eye chakra) is a deeply meditative and spiritual oil and clearing the client's third eye chakra to help channel in connection to intuition was highly beneficial for this client as they began to navigate perimenopause.
>
> Fragonia (*Taxandria fragrans*), is both emotionally and physically clearing, and using this oil on the throat chakra felt most appropriate considering the client has asthma. Channelling energy into this area can aid the client's ability to 'speak her truth' as she navigates the trauma and her changing body, mind and soul.

Rosewood was used for the heart chakra which relates to self-love and compassion. Elaine acknowledged that this is an unsustainable essential oil. She happened to have some, but she mentioned that Ho wood (*Cinnamomum camphora ct. linalool*) would be a good, sustainable replacement.

For the solar plexus chakra, Elaine used Curry leaf (*Murraya koenigii*). Her client also had irritable bowel syndrome and Elaine mentioned that she used it for its carminative, calming, antispasmodic impact and to 'channel in more energy for self-esteem and to help calm the digestive system, which is disrupted in times of trauma'.

For the sacral chakra (associated with sexuality and creativity), she used Petitgrain mandarin (*Citrus reticulata*). She told me, 'It is a powerful emotionally calming and balancing oil and using it to connect with the nurturing mother energy of the sacral chakra allowed me to channel in all that important creative energy.'

What of the root chakra, which Elaine told me is associated with root, grounding, survival, being and family? Elaine said:

> Nagarmotha (*Cyperus scariosus*) is perfectly synergetic with the root chakra. The deep, earthy animalistic scent is powerfully grounding, bringing stillness and simplicity into the body and mind. As it helps to slow the breath and calm, I also used it in the client's portable nasal inhaler.

In week one, Elaine's client arrived visibly shaking and tearful. Elaine explained that this was a safe confidential space, and showed her the different blankets and pillows she could choose from to make herself comfortable. She chose a heated blanket as it was a cold day. Elaine explained the sounds she might hear throughout the session, both inside the room and in the adjoining business properties. She demonstrated on herself how she would place her hands above or sometimes on the body (depending on appropriateness), checking out what felt comfortable with her client. She said she may move quickly or linger in areas and that her client may feel a release of energy, and she explained the possible responses that may occur. She asked her client if she had any questions and let her client know that if she felt uncomfortable at any time she could stop and Elaine would make her a cup of herbal tea.

Once her client was warmly snuggled on the couch, Elaine guided her through a grounding meditation. As she worked her heart chakra, her client released a lot of tears and Elaine checked out if it was okay to continue. Her client said it was and then started to laugh. As Elaine moved down her body, her client slowed her breathing. At the end of the session, Elaine suggested she wiggle her fingers and toes. Elaine made her a cup of herbal tea. She stayed in the treatment room for a little while afterwards, to give her a little time before having to drive home. She took home a chakra oil to aid sleep (it was 1ml with 4 drops of high-altitude Lavender (she would only use one drop of this).

Elaine would normally cleanse the room by smoking/smudging but she did not do this as her client was asthmatic (for this reason, she also avoided essential oils with high levels of 1,8-cineole). Instead, she used a hydrosol of Palo santo (*Bursera graveolens*).

In week two, Elaine's client was smiley and quite overexcited when she arrived. Elaine noted she was radically different. She had looked forward to her counselling session and felt she was making progress, and she had found the Lavender blend useful.

Elaine didn't need to explain things so much so could spend longer on this treatment and she used different essential oils this time and spent more time on the throat chakra and solar plexus. Her oil choices included Pink pepper (*Schinus molle*), which her client really connected with and was the diluted essential oil that she took home in her 1ml bottle. Her client was still experiencing sleep issues and nightmares, so Elaine gave her a sleep oil blend which she was going to use in her diffuser at home. As she was struggling to find time to use her bath salts, Elaine reminded her that even five or ten minutes sitting in half a bath of water would be better than not doing it at all.

In week three, Elaine's client arrived a little tearful after her counselling session. This week she had a big release connected to her sacral chakra. Her take-home oil was a diluted Vetiver (*Chrysopogon zizanioides*) essential oil and Elaine showed her a meditation to use with the oil.

In week four, Elaine's client really connected with Cedarwood (*Cedrus atlantica*), which was her take-home pre-diluted essential oil. Elaine also made her a grounding body oil of Ho wood and Cedarwood, with a tiny bit of Eucalyptus (*Eucalyptus globulus*).

Her client had finished her counselling sessions and had been offered occasional 'top-up' sessions with her counsellor if needed. Elaine gave her a free calendar so she could track both her menstrual cycle and her emotions. By tracking and making notes, she would be able to recognize patterns and see if it was indicating that she might need to have further counselling or reiki on her healing path, or return to her doctor. They discussed her staying in contact with her doctor and to contact the doctor if she was having any symptoms from her antidepressants. Her client had a small collection of oils at home which she continued to use and started to explore their use with other family members too.

I asked Elaine about her aromatic reiki and Elaine explained that she asks her clients to come with a question (they do not need to share this).

She uses a separate essential oil for each chakra. At the end of the session the residue of the oil is massaged into the feet, hands and scalp. While Elaine sees these two modalities as very separate, she feels they are also perfectly aligned and sometimes she includes crystals in her sessions. Elaine pointed out that while working with energy can feel quite strange to some people, she had noticed that many complementary therapists are aware of their client's energy.

Silently managing trauma

Many of us have found that clients have histories of trauma we know nothing about, or that they have silently struggled with overwhelming pain for years. UK clinical aromatherapist Sue Jenkins told me:

> I have worked for many years in private practice and have come across lots of patients experiencing or having experienced trauma of both a physical and mental nature. However, this is often not being recognized by their primary caregivers, and certainly not formalized by a diagnosis of PTSD. Many have not even consulted their doctor but have used over-the-counter medications to deal with symptoms such as insomnia, panic attacks and so forth.
>
> I have found that one of the most important tools, aside from caring touch and essential oils, is a listening ear and patience. For example, I had a client who had been coming to me for treatment for some months for general stress-related symptoms of a hectic lifestyle. She only disclosed that she had been in a dramatic air crash which killed several members of her close family (but from which she escaped with a minor injuries) when she arrived late for her session, because her daughter had been ill and sent home from school. There were floods of tears and an outpouring of grief and guilt that she had survived, and her then husband and child had not.
>
> It had taken many years for her to feel she could share her feelings. I had wondered why she was still consulting with me when her original reasons for attending had dissipated, but I was happy to continue to see her if she felt she needed the sessions. Soon after that episode she ceased her appointments, saying that the release she had felt after that one session had been enough to free herself from the trauma.

I have had many similar situations, often with older clients who will divulge traumatic childhoods, often only after years of working with them. Like Leigh, who came to me initially for aromatherapy massage at the suggestion of her doctor. As she has now known me for years, she has more recently started to share some information about her upbringing, and how she sees a connection between this and her chronic fatigue/ME. Gabor Maté gives multiple examples of where he has seen patients with autoimmune and other long-term medical conditions who have had traumatic upbringings, and we explored this in Chapter 4 (Maté, 2019; Maté & Maté, 2023).

Leigh has taught me some interesting things. For example, I have found that I had to be very careful which essential oils I use with her, sticking to a few that are solidly grounding and nurturing, typically using 0.5–1% maximum. The continuity of the same small pool of essential oils we work with helps her feel safe and in control. Essential oils that create positive change too quickly are often too much for her. I have found that some clients who are particularly sensitive can experience rapid emotional shifts with certain essential oils. While this can lead to feeling great (and for some almost euphoric) initially, the dip afterwards as it wears off can feel unpleasant. Coming 'back down to earth' feels harder when you experience fatigue.

I always used to say that a third of my clients come because of a problem that's impacting daily life, such as a stiff neck or pain in between the shoulder blades. On face value, this is normally connected to pain and often posture related due to sitting at a desk for long periods of time, but there may be other underlying issues. One third of clients come for 'maintenance' as they see the long-term physical and mental health benefits, and some are working in jobs that are quite stressful.

Another third come at a crisis point in their life when they are experiencing a high level of upset, change, trauma and distress. There may have been a recent bereavement, a relationship breakup/separation or divorce, problems with ageing parents (that often make people reflect on the relationship they have had with their parents). These clients, like Sue's clients, will often come as they work through the experience, and when they are done, they move on.

Yet what I begin to see, the more I practice, is fluidity between these three groups. Over time, some clients disclose information that gives clues about their current health, behaviours and trauma histories, not I hasten to add because I asked, but more because I was a regular part of their lives, and the time in my treatment room is safe, 'held space'.

I have lost count of the times I have heard, 'Can I tell you something' or, 'I know I can say this to you because…' Sometimes my confidentiality code needs to be repeated at this point, so they are aware of the boundaries and expectations, and to ensure we both feel safe. Sometimes parts of the puzzle start to fit together after such disclosures and, as such, the essential oils I use in the future and my approach might change.

The examples given in this chapter are from case studies and the Zoom interviews I had with many of the aromatherapists. These would be classed as qualitative in nature, and much of our 'evidence' is at times anecdotal. However, I believe they offer a rich range of aromatherapists' experience in a variety of settings.

As aromatherapists, what we see, and feel, is that essential oils help people to 'open up', to feel and listen to what resonates in their body. If you ever do an introduction to aromatherapy workshop you will see how the atmosphere in the room changes when people start smelling the essential oils. The volume of discussion often increases, people laugh, their body language becomes more open and expansive, people tell you stories about smells. The energy in the room literally changes. Therefore, as you reflect on these aromatherapists recounting their experiences and wisdom, I hope you feel as inspired and as in awe as I do. Aroma can certainly be a powerful support in people's trauma journeys.

Reflection points

- What benefits can aromatherapy services and products offer people who are traumatized?
- Have there been any common themes across these case studies?
- What aromas are culturally familiar to you?
- If you are an aromatherapist or other complementary therapist and have experience of working with people who have endured trauma, can you share this experience in a journal, so others can learn from this?

CHAPTER 8

Essential oils for trauma

For readers who are not trained in aromatherapy it is important to understand a bit about essential oils and other aromatics and how to use them safely. It is always worth reading a couple of good 'introduction to aromatherapy' texts and to research the subject before using them.

There is a lot of misinformation out there, sometimes perpetuated by people who wish to sell lots of oils, or who are well meaning but not trained. There are now plenty of online and face-to-face aromatherapy schools, and many offer introduction to aromatherapy courses as well as further training that can lead to qualifications if you want to take your interest further.

For most aromatherapists, essential oils are the main 'tool' in their aromatic work kit, but hydrolats, carrier oils, infused oils and increasingly CO_2 extracts may also be used, so I have included some information on these too.

Essential oils

There is a temptation to think that because something is natural, it is 'safe' to use in any way you wish. This is simply not true. We understand that essential oils are made up of numerous naturally occurring chemicals. Some of these indicate that we may need caution with certain essential oils or some groups of people using them. For example, we may need to use that essential oil for only a very short amount of time, use it via inhalation only or use it in much larger dilution than we would normally.

Some essential oils should be avoided during pregnancy (such as Rosemary (*Salvia Rosmarinus*), Peppermint (*Mentha x piperita*), Fennel (*Foeniculum vulgare var. dulce*), Hyssop (*Hyssopus officinalis*) and Yarrow (*Achillea millefolium*)) (Mojay, 1997) and breastfeeding. Clinically evidenced essential oils for pregnancy include Bergamot (*Citrus bergamia/*

Citrus aurantium ssp. bergamia), Lavender (*Lavandula angustifolia*), Lemon (*Citrus limonum*), Neroli (*Citrus x aurantium*) and Petitgrain (*Citrus x aurantium*) (Conrad, 2019). There are also some essential oils that should be avoided by everyone due to their toxicity.

So, what are essential oils? They are naturally derived, volatile substances that exist in many aromatic plants. They may be found in different parts of the plants, such as the seeds, roots, rhizomes, leaves, flowers, fruit rind, resin and wood. Sometimes even the whole plant contains essential oils. They are extracted via a variety of methods. Steam or water (hydro) distillation is still the most common method. Essential oils may also be extracted using expression (which typically occurs with citrus essential oils) or solvent extraction. Contrary to the name, they are not oily.

Safety first

Essential oils can be inhaled, or diluted and applied topically (e.g. placed in a carrier oil and applied to the body). We dilute them topically because they are highly concentrated and we wish to avoid adverse effects such as skin irritation. If you have seen photographs of these adverse skin reactions you will notice that they often look like chemical burns and cause a lot of pain and discomfort and can cause repeated allergies to other products you may use in the future.

Essential oils should not be ingested. Do not put them in food or drink, or use them internally (unless on the advice of a fully trained and qualified specialist advanced aromatherapist). It is especially important to make sure undiluted essential oils do not come into contact with the eyes, mouth, nose or sensitive skin such as the face and neck (Conrad, 2019).

When we dilute essential oils, we normally do this in a carrier oil (e.g. Sweet almond oil or Sunflower oil), white lotion or cream base. It needs to be oil based as essential oils do not mix with water. You should not drop them directly into a bath as they will float on the surface. Instead, mix them into a base bath or shower gel or oil or into some carrier oil which you then mix and add to Epsom or Himalayan salts.

Who can use essential oils?

Some groups of people may need to avoid certain essential oils. Some essential oils can interact with medication so, if you are taking medication, or if you have a medical condition such as epilepsy, a hormone-related cancer, blood pressure issues and so on, please consult with a trained aromatherapist first.

Children and those taking lots of medication, or people with sensitive or thinner skin, will need greater dilution. Use caution and go carefully with people who are vulnerable and cannot easily communicate their smell preference (e.g. the very sick, infirm and people with learning difficulties). Watch how they respond to an aroma before leaving it with them. Make sure you place a small drop on a tissue or smelling strip and gently waft it near them. Assess what clues they give you. Turning or pulling away, grimacing or making an unhappy noise will all suggest they are unhappy. Grinning, closed eyes flickering, lips being licked, happy sounding noises or coming towards the smell all suggest that someone likes it and is trying to smell more of it. We can observe their reactions and speak to their family and friends, who will be able to give clues about the aromas they enjoy.

Almost all essential oils should be avoided with babies and small children whose bodies are still developing. Please note, it is especially important that babies and very young children are not exposed to essential oils that contain the chemical 1,8-cineole as it can be dangerous (Tisserand & Young, 2014). 1,8-cineole may also be an irritant to some people who have asthma, though there are many essential oils that do support the respiratory system.

There are very few essential oils that we can use with very young children (under five or six years old) and it is rare to use them with children under this age. The only ones we use are normally Lavender (*Lavandula angustifolia* only), Sweet orange (*Citrus sinensis*), Roman chamomile (*Chamaemelum nobile/Anthemis nobilis*) and Mandarin (*Citrus reticulata*). I don't advocate using anything with babies and toddlers, unless you have sought advice from a qualified aromatherapist. I would normally use no more than 0.5% (1 drop of essential oil in 10ml of carrier oil) with a child under 12 years old. Most essential oils should be avoided in pregnancy and during breastfeeding.

Pets

Be aware that pets can sometimes be negatively affected by essential oils, especially Tea tree (*Melaleuca alternifolia*). This is especially true for cats who cannot easily tolerate essential oils and have very sensitive livers (Tisserand & Young, 2014). If you are using a diffuser, always leave the door open so they are free to leave the room, remember to ventilate well, and do not use for long periods of time. Do not use essential oils directly on animals unless you have undergone specific training in using aromatherapy with animals from a qualified specialist aromatherapist.

Buying and storing essential oils

Only buy essential oils in dark glass bottles as sunlight can degrade them. Always ensure you buy ones that have the Latin name and country of origin on them, and have droppers inserted so you can safely use them. Please buy them from a reputable source that sells ethical and sustainable essential oils. I prefer to use organic or wild-crafted essential oils where possible. The Airmid Institute[1] produces a free biannual list of essential oil producing plants that have sustainability issues. I always recommend consulting this, as many essential oils come from endangered plants.

Keep your essential oils in a cool, dark environment, the lids tightly secured, away from children and pets (along with other things associated with essential oil use like diffusers). Citrus and Pine essential oils shouldn't be kept for more than nine months. Other essential oils can generally be kept for two years, although some can be kept for longer. Your supplier should be able to verify how long your essential oil purchases should be kept for.

Topical use

There are many carrier oils you can use, which have their own amazing properties. If you have a nut allergy, you will want to use carrier oils like sunflower seed oil or grapeseed oil. Please note that certain essential oils are not indicated for topical use or should only be used in very small amounts (e.g. 0.5% of essential oil to 99.5% of carrier oil). Always research each essential oil before you use it and if in doubt always ask a qualified aromatherapist.

Depending on the age and weight of a teenager, you may use an adult dilution for those over 12 years old, but some aromatherapists recommend adult dilutions to be used at 16 years and above (Tisserand & Young, 2014). Please note that because a drop will differ in size (and weight) due to several variables, such as the viscosity of the oil or the

---

1   https://airmidinstitute.org

dropper, you will sometimes see variations in the number of drops and the percentage dilution this equates to.

For example, 2.5 drops per 5ml of carrier oil or 5 drops per 10ml of carrier oil (Kerkhof, 2023) may be considered as a 2% blend. This is based on an average of 25 drops of essential oil in 1ml (Kerkhof, 2023).

As it is tricky to measure 2.5 drops in 5ml, some round up or down, for example 3 drops to 5ml of carrier oil or 6 drops to 10ml of carrier oil (Tisserand & Young, 2014). I tend to round down and use 2 drops in 5ml or 4–5 drops in 10ml. For those taking medication, reduce this to 1% dilution (2 drops per 10ml of carrier oil). In pregnancy, use 0.5–1% maximum (for more information, see Conrad, 2019).

I find no need to go above 2% when I am using essential oils for emotional, psychological or spiritual use and will sometimes use only 1% in these instances (1 drop per 5ml of carrier oil or 2 drops per 10ml of carrier oil). Some clients who have experienced trauma are especially sensitive to the subtle energetics of the essential oil and as such a much lower amount, such as 1% (or even 0.5%), may be desirable.

Inhalation

If you wish to inhale essential oils, this can easily be achieved through one of the following methods.

Diffuser

Add water to the fill line on your electric diffuser reservoir. Then add a few drops of essential oil. You don't need to diffuse for more than 30 minutes. I suggest then leaving it for a few hours before turning it back on. Do not diffuse essential oils for hours and do not sit right next to an essential oil diffuser. Be aware of other people in the setting who may not like the aroma, may get a reaction from it or could even be triggered by it.

Inhaler aroma stick

You can buy these online, and while plastic ones are available, reusable metal ones are becoming more popular. These can be placed in a pocket or bag, so are very portable. I use between 8 and 10 drops of essential oil. Put the essential oil into a small bowl or egg cup and stand the filter into it, allowing it to absorb the essential oil fully before popping it into the casing and adding the stopper. I then give mine a shake and add the outer protective cap. Label it with a sticker so you can remember the oils you have used.

Aroma patches

These can be bought pre-infused and ready to use, or blank and you can add essential oil to them. They are most popular in hospital settings and palliative care, as they can be attached to clothing.

Hydrolats/Hydrosols

These are produced when essential oils are distilled; as the steam cools the essential oil separates off from the water (which becomes the hydrolat). Although they may have been viewed as a by-product in the past, they certainly have a place in herbal medicine and aromatherapy. Water soluble constituents of the aromatic plant material are found in the water which also contains the tiniest trace elements of essential oil.

Some aromatherapists prefer to use them with younger children, especially as they are so much gentler, and we saw how Cynthia used a blend with her client who was a young child, and how Nicole uses them in Lebanon. As they are water based, they also work nicely as facial mists, pillow sprays and room sprays and can be added to products. They should be kept in a refrigerator, and you should consult your supplier for information on shelf life.

CO_2 extracts

While CO_2 extracts have been used in food and perfumery since the 1970s and 80s, they are still relatively novel for the vast majority of aromatherapists. So, what are they?

Carbon dioxide (CO_2) changes state when subjected to changes in pressure and temperature. By facilitating and harnessing this possibility, we can use CO_2 like a 'solvent' to get the beneficial compounds that we wish to remove from the plant material. The 'end product' of this is our CO_2 extract.

After this extraction has taken place, the temperature and pressure are returned to normal and the CO_2 returns to its original state. Unlike traditional solvents, nothing nasty is left behind in the material. It is very environmentally friendly (though the machinery required is very expensive). Another good thing about CO_2 extracts is that we can also obtain the benefits of plants that we normally think of as base oils, such as Evening primrose oil. For more information on these, I suggest you read *CO_2 Extracts in Aromatherapy* by Madeleine Kerkhof (2018). She is an expert in CO_2 extracts and has working tirelessly to increase awareness of them in the aromatherapy community.

Although CO_2 extracts contain some essential oils they are not the same as essential oils, as their chemical makeup demonstrates. There are three different types of CO_2 extract available – select extract, sub CO_2 extract and total extract. These three types come about through differing amounts of pressure and temperature change. Selects look (and are used) rather like essential oils. Total extracts contain waxes, fats, pigments and so on, as these are CO_2 soluble. Totals are often thicker/gloopy and may need to be warmed before using.

Carrier/Base oils or infused/macerated oils

Carrier (or base) oils are often called vegetable oils and tend to come from nuts, seeds or kernels of plants. Examples include Sweet almond, Sunflower, Grapeseed, Coconut, Jojoba or Wheatgerm oils. Sometimes a carrier oil (such as Sunflower oil) has been infused with a medicinal plant (such as Arnica, St Johns or Calendula oil).

Aromatherapy choices

In previous books, I have included formulas for aromatherapeutic blends and products. I do not believe it would be appropriate for me to do so here as our smell preferences are so personal, and we understand how easily aroma can be a trigger. When I asked US aromatherapist Rehne Burge (who specializes in working with people who have experienced trauma and PTSD) what advice she would give to other aromatherapists she told me, 'One solution cannot accommodate all clients. Trauma is one's own personal experience(s).'

So, we must always remember that the *personal* meaning of a smell is of particular importance when working with trauma. I think it is up to the individual aromatherapist to choose to offer a single oil or blend depending on the client's goal, how they are working together and what the client is experiencing.

Symptoms of trauma, as we have seen, can be so wide ranging. How I work, and the essential oils I choose to use with a client in their seventies who has chronic pain from an autoimmune condition (which has possibly come from the damage to their immune system during their childhood experience of neglect and abuse), may be very different from what I would do with someone who is presenting with a recent PTSD diagnosis, who is hypersensitive to touch, hyperaroused, has serious sleep deprivation, flashbacks and has been triggered several times in the week before coming to see me. It is about understanding what our clients need and following their lead, rather than following a prescribed blend in a book. After all, this is what makes aromatherapy holistic.

If you are a qualified aromatherapist reading this, I encourage you to use your knowledge but also your intuition. What do you see and 'feel' in your client? Carefully following your client's reaction to a single essential oil or blend that you use is essential.

Scientific research tends to use a single essential oil. This makes sense as it makes it easier to isolate what works and what doesn't. It lessens the variables that could intervene and narrows down the pharmaceutical providence of the naturally occurring chemical constituents. For example, if a blend created a reaction, it would be hard to know if that was due to the entire blend or one single oil or a particular chemical component. As aromatherapists, we often use blends that lend themselves to creating a harmonious synergy. There are advantages to this as well. For example, Langley-Brady *et al.* (2023) note that it may be most appropriate to mix a blend of four or more oils when doing reactive aromatherapy. They state that this is because it is hard to pick out individual chemical constituents when inhaling a blend of oils at once, and there is less likelihood of a blend being triggering (as opposed to an individual oil).

It is important, as previously mentioned, to also be aware of smell triggers. You may have to use your own knowledge of smells to avoid certain aromas. For example, I detect a slight whiff of a fuel-like odour in certain essential oils such as some Frankincense (*Boswellia carteri*), Copal santo (*Bursera copallifera*) and Breu Branco/Brazilian frankincense (*Protium heptaphyllum*). Given that fuel can be a smell trigger, especially with those who have worked in combat zones, or experienced aviation or automobile accidents, it would be worth avoiding these, especially in single use. If someone has a positive memory of Frankincense (e.g. for religious reasons), that might change your decision.

If you know the context of someone's trauma it may help you to distinguish what not to use, but we must always be prepared for the fact that sometimes we (and even they) do not have this information.

I do not have an exhaustive list of essential oils, carrier oils, CO_2s and hydrolats I would use for trauma, but I do acknowledge that there are several essential oils, hydrolats and other aromatics that kept coming up in conversations with aromatherapists or in the research. There are certainly ones that lend themselves to certain aspects of living with trauma.

I have chosen to profile just some of these and illuminate their usefulness. I have also included other properties so you can see if you feel this is appropriate depending on what someone is presenting with on the day. You may have several others you would like to add.

ESSENTIAL OILS

Angelica root (*Angelica archangelica*)

In history, Angelica has often been thought to be a highly protective plant, warding off both disease and evil (Bhat, Kumar & Shah, 2011). It belongs to the family Apiaceae and has essential oil in its seeds, roots, stem and leaves.

Physically, it is deemed to be useful for digestive issues and motion sickness and it has carminative properties. It may be helpful for joint or muscle pain as it is anti-inflammatory. It is also indicated for respiratory issues, congestion which is hard to resolve, and physical weakness (Nagle-Smith, 2024), and has antibacterial and antifungal properties (Rhind, 2020).

It is an energetically warming and drying essential oil (Battaglia, 2018). Fischer-Rizzi (1990) describes it as being useful for times when it is hard to make decisions, or your perseverance needs increasing. Warner (2018) recommends it for times when people feel afraid and traumatized, and Skipper (2022) recommends it for dissociation and those who need to be more present and grounded. She says of it:

> It fills the spiritual body with a golden light and hugs the heart. It has a deeply calming resonance that helps relieve anxious states and supports people struggling with PTSD. Gently reminding us that we are loved, and that negative thought patterns, emotions and self-doubt aren't who we truly are. (Skipper, 2019)

Cautions

This is a phototoxic essential oil. Tisserand and Young (2014) suggest that using more than 0.8% poses a risk of phototoxicity (so sunlight and sunbeds should be avoided for 12 hours). They cite Rudski *et al.* (1976), who carried out a study of 200 dermatitis patients and found that 1% of them were sensitive to 2% dermal application of the essential oil. Aromatherapists would be unlikely to use as much as a 2% dilution of essential oil in carrier oil if they knew a client had sensitive skin. I would not use more than 0.5% of Angelica root essential oil in a carrier oil, and I would avoid it with those with sensitive skin. Diabetics should also avoid it as it might alter sugar levels (Bhat *et al.*, 2011). Avoid if pregnant or breastfeeding.

Australian rosewood (*Dysoxylum fraserianum*)

First, this should not be mistaken for Rosewood (*Aniba rosaeodora*), which is a completely different tree and is endangered. The Australian rosewood tree is from the family Meliaceae and is native to New South Wales, Australia, and doesn't seem to be widely used beyond that country. It was assessed by the International Union for Conservation of Nature (IUCN) Red List in 2020 and is marked as being of 'least concern' (IUCN Red List, 2020).

To date, I have been using an essential oil that is obtained by steam distillation of the leaves and green branchlets from trees purposefully grown on a plantation (Essentially Australia, 2023). I believe there are suppliers who also provide it from aged timber that has fallen by its own volition or been left behind from past decades of logging (as it doesn't decompose like other woods) (Native Extracts, 2023). The essential oil is a beautiful blue colour and as soon as I started to use it, I knew it was special.

The oil contains several sesquiterpenes, and Australian growers and sellers indicate it for skin conditions (which in my anecdotal experience often get worse or start during trauma) and calming the mind and emotions. However, there is barely any information on it, as it is such a new essential oil.

It smells like Sandalwood, possibly lighter and a bit floral. It can easily get lost in a blend, but I have found it tremendously useful for those who are feeling sad, alone or traumatized or who are grieving. It seems to soothe the heart and soul, bringing a real sense of peace, stillness and serenity to everyone I have used it with. It also seems to pacify the mind. Unlike Indian sandalwood (*Santalum album*) or Australian sandalwood (*Santalum spicatum*) there are no sustainability issues. I now tend to use it in place of Sandalwood, and it is one of my 'go to' essential oils for trauma, grief and heartache.

Cautions

Australian rosewood is a very new essential oil on the aromatherapy market, and at the time of writing, and to my knowledge, there is nothing published on this, so we do not have safety data.

Bergamot (*Citrus bergamia/Citrus aurantium ssp. bergamia*)

Bergamot is a popular, easy to source essential oil from the family Rutaceae and is derived from the rind of the fruit. With its fresh citrus, almost slightly floral aroma it is generally loved, and I have never met anyone who does not like the smell. It has been used in several PTSD studies with humans, so is starting to slowly develop a clinical evidence base.

It is antidepressant and anxiolytic (meaning it is used to reduce anxiety) (Lizarraga-Valderrama, 2023). Bergamot is also mood enhancing, immune supporting, wound healing and antinociceptive (so it can help with reducing feelings of pain) (Rhind, 2020). Rhind (2020) notes that there is an evidence base illustrating the usefulness of Bergamot essential oils in reducing heart rate and blood pressure, anxiety and stress, pain and depression. She unpacks this on an even deeper level by pointing to research by Morrone *et al.* (2007) that indicates potential release of amino acids in the hippocampus, which act as neurotransmitters and impact synaptic plasticity (which is thought to contribute to memory and learning). She then tells us, 'This suggests an activation of olfactory-hippocampal pathways, a premise supported by Saiyudthong and Marsden (2011), who proposed that Bergamot can attenuate hypothalamic-pituitary-adrenal activity by reducing the corticosterone response to stressors' (Rhind, 2020, p.571).

Daniel and Zolnikov (2023) carried out a two-week qualitative pilot study with 12 men and women who had PTSD. Participants were asked to inhale the essential oil by placing 2 drops of an essential oil directly on the hands (though I would caution against this due to the possibility of phototoxicity and sensitization) and sniffing three times a day at allotted times. They were then asked to use it in a diffuser in the bedroom at night, and to record their experiences in a journal. There were many positive outcomes, including improved sleep, reduced anxiety, fewer angry outbursts, avoidance behaviours and panic attacks (reduced both in occurrence and length) and increased positive mood.

The authors state that they chose Bergamot because existing research showed it reduced heart rate, modulated various neurotransmitters involved in PTSD and had a calming action on the neuroendocrine system. Many participants talked of feeling calmer, one forgot their attention deficit hyperactivity disorder (ADHD) medication but still felt attentive and clear headed, others talked about their head or their thoughts being in a better place. Interestingly, two participants reported finding it easier to talk to someone about their feelings or past trauma (Daniel & Zolnikov, 2023). Emerald (2016) also points to research that demonstrates its potential for PTSD. Eastholm (2018) also used Bergamot in a blend with war veterans who had PTSD. She cites Watanabe *et al.* (2015) for this rationale, noting that they had found participants' heart rates had improved and their cortisol levels were lowered.

On a subtle level, Bosson (2019) states it adds joy to life, eliminating bitterness, anxieties and worry about existential questions. Kerkhof (2023) also tells us that when there are existential questions, Bergamot helps us not to sink into darkness. I have found in my clinical use it is extremely helpful for anger, frustration, paranoia and feelings of being judged, as well as feelings of 'no one gets me/understands'. Both can lead to a sense of 'otherness' and separation that can come from feeling as if everyone else is leading a normal life and you aren't. Bosson recommends using the hydrosol as a spray for the aura or drinking a teaspoon of the hydrosol in water two to three times a day.

Holmes (2016) tells us that in Traditional Chinese Medicine, Bergamot regulates the Qi energy and harmonizes the shen. He notes it is extremely useful for times when symptoms swing between hyper- and hypo-functioning. He also indicates it for addictive behaviours, insomnia, negative thoughts patterns and situations where balance and harmony are required. Guthrie states, 'Its ability to regulate the autonomic nervous system makes it a wonderful ally when a person is working to expand their spectrum of tolerance' (Guthrie, 2023, p.73).

This makes it useful if we want to support people in increasing their ability to express their emotions and move beyond existing self-dialogue and coping mechanisms. Bergamot has the character of a friendly person who will always be happy to see you, taking your hand and encouraging you to step out of your comfort zone.

Cautions

Bergamot is phototoxic due to the furocoumarin content. As such, it should not be used on areas of skin where there is going to be contact with direct sunlight nor should it be used for up to 12 hours before going on a sunbed. It is possible to buy Bergamot without this content (it is called Bergamot FCF). If you are not using Bergamot FCF then suggested dermal use (i.e. on the skin) is limited to 0.4% (Tisserand & Young, 2014) due to the risk of phototoxicity, and it should be kept in a refrigerator.

Cedarwood atlas (*Cedrus atlantica*)

Cedars are huge, beautiful trees that produce the most amazing essential oil (which comes from the distillation of wood chips and sawdust). They belong to the family Pinaceae. Cedarwood atlas has a warm, sweet woody aroma and is now sadly endangered, so we have to question whether we should even be using it, and if we do so then we should use it sparingly (IUCN Red List, 2023). Cedarwood virgina (*Juniperus virginiana*) is often suggested as an alternative because the aroma is quite similar, but it should be noted that this is actually a Juniper and its actions, chemistry and effects will differ. Nicole's experience in Chapter 7 demonstrates how it is a culturally important and familiar tree in Lebanon.

The essential oil has analgesic, anti-inflammatory and sedative properties and may be used for the respiratory system, and problems with the skin (Rhind, 2020). I find it helpful in blends for eczema that gets worse in times of distress.

On a spiritual and emotional level, Cedarwood provides tremendous support and strength, holding you steady in turbulent times, especially where there is fear or overwhelm. I have used it a lot with clients who need to hold steady in the moment and just take things one step at a time. It seems to reduce overthinking and allows someone to catch their emotional breath so they can be calm and manage things.

Warner (2018) says it is one of the most spiritually grounding essential oils and that it provides warmth, strength and courage, while Holmes (2016) suggests it for people who experience dissociation, disconnection and repetitive thinking as well as for those who feel fearful, unsafe, insecure or unable to let go.

Guthrie (2023) recommends using it with Bergamot (*Citrus bergamia/ Citrus aurantium ssp. bergamia*) and Grapefruit (*Citrus paradisi*) for a dorsal vagal-inspired blend. I like to blend it with Bergamot, Neroli (*Citrus x aurantium*) or Rose (*Rosa damascena*) in particular.

Cautions

There are no known contraindications or hazards (Tisserand & Young, 2014).

Cistus (*Cistus ladaniferus*)

Cistus is also known as Rockrose. It comes from the family Cistaceae and is an aromatic shrub that grows in the Mediterranean. Its aroma has been described in many ways, with words such as warm, dry, sweet and woody being common. I have also seen people add the words musky, slightly spicy, floral and earthy to the mix.

The plant can produce two essential oils. One is Cistus oil (obtained from the steam distillation of the whole flowering plant. The other is Labdanum, which is produced from the gum (Tisserand & Young, 2014). Some authors do not distinguish which they are talking about when discussing the plant.

It is antioxidant, antitumoral, anti-inflammatory, antimicrobial, antifungal, antidepressant, antispasmodic and antihypertensive. Rhind (2020) states that many internet and commercial websites cite it as useful for trauma. Purchon and Cantele (2014) state it has a sedative action on the nervous system and is useful for chronic fatigue, fibromyalgia, anxiety and insomnia.

Energetically, Fischer-Rizzi (1990) says it is yang in nature, and useful for the soul, helping those who feel cold, empty, numb or shaky following trauma. She says it calms, centres and brings a sense of consciousness.

Cautions
Tisserand and Young (2014) note it may cause skin irritation if the essential oil is oxidized. If it is used in products they recommend adding an antioxidant.

Copaiba (*Copaifera officinalis*)
Copaiba essential oil is distilled from the oleoresin of the tree. Aromatherapists can also use the oleoresin like an essential oil too (it is slightly thicker and has diterpenes which give extra benefit if using it for skin healing). I have previously found little written about it, so I have summarized some of the information from my previous book (Nagle-Smith, 2024).

Like many trees from the family Burseraceae, it may also be known as Copal, and it is from the family Leguminosae, sub-family Detarioideae (sometimes also known as Fabaceae, sub-family Detarioideae). Traditional use includes healing respiratory issues, wounds and infections and managing pain or skin problems, smudging or ceremonial use to banish evil spirits (Nagle-Smith, 2024). It is spasmolytic, sedative, antibacterial and antiviral. It can be useful in pain blends due to its naturally occurring beta-caryophyllene having cannabimimetic effects, hence it is neuroprotective, anti-inflammatory and antinociceptive (Rhind, 2020). I do not do scar reduction work but for those aromatherapists who do incorporate this, it would be worth considering adding Copaiba oleo-resin to your repertoire. It is already used in some commercial brands of cream for this purpose (Waibel *et al.*, 2021). While it can work on physical scars, it is also useful for emotional wounds.

I use it in my clinical work where there is nerve pain (e.g. especially after shocking or traumatic accidents). Quietly powerful, it is 'a calm healer for deep-seated wounds, unspoken hurt and emotional trauma' (Nagle-Smith, 2024, p.78).

Brazilian aromatherapist Carla Véscovi specializes in teaching about essential oils native to Brazil and she was the person who taught me how important Copaiba is, showing me that this is a great facilitator, helping people to 'let go' (Nagle-Smith, 2024). I have found it especially supportive where there are things that people find hard to voice, or they feel they can't talk openly about. I have used it a lot for physical issues that affect the more private areas of our body. For example, I have used it heavily diluted at 1% maximum in a carrier oil for haemorrhoids or perineum scarring. You could start with 0.5% first to assess its suitability. Sometimes, issues with the skin, sensation, or fear of touch in this area can occur as the result of a traumatic birth and as such the Copaiba can work on the physical and mental aspects of this. The gentle application can be controlled by the client and can help them reconnect to their body.

Changes to the body due to ageing, illness or perimenopause, unwanted touch or abuse, medical examinations, feeling that you are in the wrong body, surgery, toxic relationships and sexual grief are just a few of the many reasons that people feel uncomfortable, shameful, embarrassed about or disassociated from the more private parts of their body.

For instance, where there has been old scar tissue in the area I have used a blend of 2 drops of pre-diluted Rose (*Rosa damascena*) essential oil (I use one that is pre-diluted in 90% Jojoba oil (*Simmondsia chinensis*)) and 1 drop of Copaiba oleoresin to 10ml of Coconut oil (*Cocos nucifera*). Coconut oil is particularly moisturizing and protective. It has antibacterial and anti-itching properties (Kerkhof 2023). You will need to gently melt it in a bain-marie first and then put the Rose and Copaiba in and stir. Once hardened, a pea-sized amount can be used. I suggest people put this in the palm of one clean hand and let it melt with the heat of the hand and then apply it with a clean finger. Alternatively, I have found Sweet almond oil is quite useful as it never feels too greasy and seems to dry quicker, thus making people more inclined to use it.

Sometimes even the concept of touching that part of the body with the scars or dryness is too much and if this is the case, I would suggest the person may wish to just focus on light sweeping strokes on the outside of their thigh, moving over a period of days or weeks (if they feel okay with this) to the inside of their thigh, or buttocks. Very gradually, they can build up their ability to manage self-touch in this area of their body.

Cautions
I have seen it referred to as being a potential skin irritant by aromatherapy authors, which may be because it contains large amounts of beta-caryophyllene (just like Black pepper (*Piper nigrum*)). Tisserand (2017) notes that despite this popular belief, it is not a skin irritant. Tisserand and Young (2014) tell us that in one test it caused irritation to rabbits but with a test on 25 humans at 8% (which is way higher than I would ever be using) no sensitization was found (Tisserand, 2017).

Everlasting/Immortelle/Helichrysum (*Helichrysum italicum*)
Everlasting belongs to the family Asteraceae and the essential oil is derived from steam distillation of the flowering head. The plant grows in the Mediterranean and has a warm, slightly spicy, sweet aroma.

Rhind (2020) says there is no such thing as a 'typical' composition and its chemical makeup differs depending on the area it is grown in. Aromatherapists should therefore check the GC-MS (gas chromatography/mass spectrometry) before making their choice. A good essential oil supplier would be able to send you this, or have it available on their website. Rhind (2020) notes its main actions are being analgesic, anti-inflammatory, antibacterial, wound healing and anti-hematomal, as well as being useful for allergic responses. Everlasting is often used in trauma blends for physical trauma where there may be bruising and swelling, but aromatherapists also consider it useful for emotional or soul wounds.

When it comes to PTSD, it is not an essential oil that would readily be found in research papers, yet among aromatherapists it has become increasingly popular over the last 30–40 years, and many tell me that they use it for deep-seated wounds and things deep in the psyche.

Elizabeth Ashley (2016, p.77) calls it 'the essential oil for wounds that will not heal' and she doesn't mean just physical ones. Ashley (2016) quotes Worwood, who told us this was an essential oil for people with deep-seated painful emotions who find it painfully impossible to bring these up, and for the walking wounded. This theme is continued in the work of other aromatherapists.

Bosson (2019) recommends the hydrosol for people who want to move on from a difficult childhood, purify their past and move forwards with serenity.

Ashley notes how it has been indicated for addiction and trauma and how this makes sense to her. She tells us:

> When I first picked up the oil I could see war, perhaps it was the vibration of the war that has so recently scarred Croatia that I saw. I could smell the dirt, the blood, the stench of fear. The darkness was obliterated by the brightness of fire and explosions rang in my ears. Most certainly this is a medicine for the traumatized and the numbed. (Ashley, 2016, p.97)

Cathy Skipper writes:

> Its wound healing properties bring disconnected parts of ourselves back together to be held at a central point of alignment. This is ideal when identifying and incorporating transgenerational trauma. Helichrysum helps us clear the fears that act as blockages to feeling and opening the whole of ourselves. (Skipper, 2020a)

Kerkhof (2023) says that this essential oil provides warm support, comfort, peace, and fresh courage during crisis and trauma. Davis (2005, p.141) refers to it as 'honey for the psyche', which for me sums up everything I read about its esoteric qualities.

Cautions
There is the possibility that it may interfere with blood clotting and should therefore be avoided by those taking blood-thinning medication such as Warfarin. More research is required, but in the absence of this it is best to avoid it in these circumstances (Kerkhof, 2023). Do not use in pregnancy or during breastfeeding.

Frankincense (*Boswellia spp.*)
In aromatherapy, we use a few different types of Frankincense, including *Boswellia carteri*, *Boswellia sacra* and *Boswellia serrata*. You may also hear Frankincense referred to as Olibanum. It has a fascinating and long history of ceremonial and spiritual use. Frankincense resin is steam distilled

to produce the essential oil which has a distinctive and quite strong aroma that is often associated with churches. For some it holds great comfort and peace, but for others it can be unsettling and triggering.

The essential oil has many useful properties, including being analgesic, antinociceptive, anti-inflammatory, immune stimulating, antibacterial, antioxidant and antifungal (Rhind, 2020). I use it quite a lot for people who have long-term pain from something like arthritis (often blending it with Katafray (*Cedrelopsis grevei*), Kunzea (*Kunzea ambigua*), Lavender (*Lavandula angustifolia*), Copaiba (*Copaifera officinalis*), a Spruce, Fragonia (*Taxandria fragrans*), Everlasting (*Helichrysum italicum*), Plai (*Zingiber cassumunar/Zingiber montanum*) or Brazilian pepper (*Schinus terebinthifolia*).

It is also incredibly useful for people who have hyperventilation syndrome, and who feel constriction in their chest. Many people find it helps to still the mind, calming them down and reducing overwhelm. It often seems to lift the mood and reduce worry. I find it can be quite helpful when people feel a bit restless or wired. Véscovi (2022) notes she sometimes uses it to help people expand their ability to look beyond their body and encounter their divine part, so their pain can transform into learning.

My first experience of using Frankincense was in a massage blend while a fellow trainee aromatherapist gave me an aromatherapy massage. While my friend massaged me, I saw a vivid image in my mind of a number of horses galloping along a shoreline together. In my next aromatherapy massage with it, I imagined I was standing underneath a deep blue cathedral ceiling painted with tiny golden stars. Both images were serene but very strong and the experience was very surreal. It unnerved me somewhat, so I steered clear of Frankincense for many months.

What I realized, years later, was that Frankincense gave me the same notion I get when I stand on a beach and look out to sea – a sense of being something very small in an amazing world. It brings a feeling of worldly connection to nature and something beyond us, it minimizes rumination and helps us appreciate what we have, letting go of fear and insecurities.

These experiences helped me comprehend that it could help those who overthink, or get caught in cyclical conversations in their head, and that it could help people think they belonged to something important and far greater. In particular, it may help with understanding that perhaps in life none of us is truly alone as we are all part of something bigger.

Fragonia® (*Taxandria fragrans*)

Fragonia is from the family Myrtaceae and has been available since 2002 (you may also see it called *Agonis fragrans*). It is a newer Australian essential oil and was brought to the aromatherapy market by the Day family, who are currently the only supplier. It has a green, lemon, slightly honey sweetness with a medicinal, 1,8-cineole aroma that runs through it, tinged by a soapy note.

It has many physical benefits for the body. It is anti-inflammatory, analgesic and antispasmodic, and as such I find it useful in pain blends; however, as it is very antibacterial, antiviral, antimicrobial and antifungal, it is good when the body's defences are down, and people fall ill with coughs, colds and viruses (which often happens in the wake of acute trauma or grief). It is also antioxidant (Nagle-Smith, 2024).

It can be an incredibly emotionally balancing, soothing essential oil and much of this is attributed to its naturally occurring chemistry (it has almost even amounts of oxides, alcohols and monoterpenes) (Nagle-Smith, 2024). Warner (2018) indicates it for times of transition. I have found it a useful oil for people who feel stuck, for example someone who feels that their illness holds them back and yet they don't seem to make any changes that could be positive. It evens out the emotions, erodes resentment and conflict and helps us move past blockages that hold us back and continue our suffering. It imbues a sense that all will be well (Nagle-Smith, 2024).

Interestingly, Dr Peneol considers it to be yin/feminine and for Kunzea (*Kunzea ambigua*) to be yang/masculine. He states that when they work in tandem, they increase the outcomes for the individual (Day, 2008). It was used alongside Kunzea and Katafray (*Cedrelopsis grevei*) in a blend following the Grenfell fire (as discussed with Jane Lawson in the previous chapter).

Cautions

Tisserand and Young (2014) cite no known ill effects. It can create skin sensitization if oxidized, so avoid keeping it for too long and store it in a dark, airtight container or fridge. Due to 1,8-cineole, there is a low risk of skin sensitization, but it is generally considered to be non-toxic (Tisserand & Young, 2014).

Galbanum (*Ferula galbaniflua*)

Galbanum essential oil is distilled from oleoresin. It is rather curious, because we normally associate oleoresin with trees from the family

Burseraceae, but Galbanum is from the family Ferula and the plant is a large perennial herb. Rhind (2020) tells us that the oleoresin is found in ducts around the plant, normally at the joints, and after a cut is made at the base or roots, the oleoresin runs down and collects there. It has been used in many cultures as incense.

Very little is written about Galbanum, but it is thought to potentially be an expectorant and to be antinociceptive, anti-inflammatory and wound healing. Traditionally, it has been used as a respiratory tonic (Rhind, 2020).

My first encounter with Galbanum was when I was getting over a chest infection. I had sore chest muscles and it felt as if my whole ribcage ached. At the time, aromatherapist Emma Pearson (who was a student then) was doing her case studies. When she told me she would like to use Galbanum in my blend I was intrigued and asked more about it. When I smelt it, I felt as if I was being punched in the face. It made me physically recoil. The smell is quite something. Very green, sharp and forceful. Rhind (2020) describes this wonderfully when she says it smells of cut green bell peppers, with piney, earthy, musty notes. It reminds me of Perilla and maybe Devils Club. Rhind suggests using Roman chamomile (*Chamaemelum nobile/Anthemis nobilis*) or Blackcurrant bud to soften the aroma if needed. I would suggest this would also soften it energetically.

Emma Pearson had investigated Galbanum in some depth and when I was struggling to write my last book and kept procrastinating, she said it was the perfect essential oil to use for this. I have found writing this book really hard and writing about trauma often difficult. A single drop of Galbanum, on a tissue in the room, helped (though I found it so strong, it couldn't be too close to me). He (it's a very masculine energy in my mind) would propel me forwards, reminding me to push through and keep writing. I explore working with it, alongside Rose (*Rosa damascena*), later in this chapter.

Rhind (2020) also suggests using it with Lavender (*Lavandula angustifolia*), Geranium (*Pelargonium x asperum*), Violet leaf (*Viola odorata*) or Hyacinth (*Hyacinthus orientalis*).

Warner (2018) writes about Galbanum as a sacred oil, saying it has a long history of being used in incense, in the Bible and by the Egyptians and Romans. She says it can teach the soul and may reveal secrets from your shadow, though she notes it is energetically very powerful when used in spiritual work and perhaps should only be used by those who are experienced in doing this work.

Cautions

Tisserand and Young (2014) note it may cause skin irritation if oxidized, so old or oxidized oils should be avoided. They state that an antioxidant should be added if it is used in products. The oil can polymerize as it ages.

Geranium (*Pelargonium x asperum*)

Belonging to the family Geraniaceae, Geranium may also be known by the Latin name *Pelargonium x asperum* (Tisserand & Young, 2014).

Rhind (2020) notes it is analgesic, anti-inflammatory, hypotensive, vasorelaxant, antifungal, antibacterial, anxiolytic and antidepressant. It is beneficial for skin conditions, soft tissue damage and oedema (and subsequent pain and inflammation). It can also assist in reducing stress, tension, anxiety and mood swings.

I have had many clients over the years who have developed oedema as a result of a disabling medical condition or an injury to their legs that was traumatic. It can sometimes be a painful, physical reminder of what they can no longer do or the traumatic incident itself.

I always think of Geranium as an emotionally balancing essential oil that calms and relieves stress. Battaglia (2018) cites Loughran and Bull (2001) who say it enables us to connect, not only with ourselves but also those around us. Guthrie (2023) suggests using it to help clients 'open the heart', when trauma shuts them off, and to reduce the need to protectively hunch over or the jumpiness that comes with hypervigilance.

Cautions

Do not use if taking diabetes medication or medication metabolized by the gene CYP2B6 (Tisserand & Young, 2014).[2]

Grapefruit (*Citrus paradisi*)

Grapefruit belongs to the family Rutaceae and the essential oil is steam distilled or expressed from the rind of the fruit. With a clean, fresh, zesty, citrus twang, it smells very familiar, though to my nose smells ever so

---

2   This could be of consequence for people taking anaesthetics (such as Ketamine, Lidocaine and propofol), antiarrhythmic medication (e.g. Mexiletine), anticoagulants, anti-convulsants, antidepressants (e.g. Bupropion), antiepileptic medication, some anti-inflammatorys, antiretroviral medication (e.g. for HIV), chemopatheraputic medications (e.g. for cancer) such as Tamoxifen, MAOI, opiods (e.g. Methadone or Pethidine), psychotropics (e.g. Diazapam, Clotiazepam, Temazepam) and steroids (e.g. Testosterone) (Hedrich, Hassan & Wang, 2016). If in doubt, do not use.

slightly sweeter than the sharp Grapefruit we would eat for breakfast on Christmas morning. It may help digestive issues, musculoskeletal problems and general well-being and is a stimulating essential oil indicated for combating fatigue and lethargy (Rhind, 2020). Holmes (2019) says it is one of the most beneficial essential oils if we want to heal the head heart connection, commenting that it carefully highlights negative thoughts, while enabling both mental and emotional clarity. It is also useful for those who get easily distracted (Holmes, 2019), which may also be why it is often used in blends to focus the mind.

Guthrie (2023) has found in her client work that it is good for providing mental uplift and moving out of mental fogginess or sluggishness and feelings of overwhelm that have built up over time. I certainly find it very helpful for mental stimulation.

Cautions

You will sometimes see it suggested not to use Grapefruit if you are using medication metabolized by the CYP3A4 enzyme (e.g. statins and anxiolytic medication) because the fruit/juice of Grapefruit can interact with the medication. Tisserand (2018), however, states that this is not the case with the essential oil because the dihydroxybergamottin is the constituent we are trying to avoid, and while it is present in grapefruit juice, it does not exist in the essential oil. Bergamottin is also thought to have a low impact, but this is a tiny amount of the essential oil and would only impact you if used internally, which would not be advisable anyway for other safety reasons. It also poses a phototoxicity risk and as such should not be used any higher than 4% according to Tisserand and Young (2014). Direct sunlight and sunbeds should be avoided for up to 12 hours after using on the skin.

Ho wood (*Cinnamomum camphora ct. linalool*)

Ho wood is a sustainable essential oil that comes from steam distilling either the wood or wood and leaves together. It has a soft floral, peppery, herbal sweet note among a light woody aroma and is generally very non-offensive. Ho wood may also be known as Ho, Ho sho, Ho shiu, Ho-leaf or Shui-sho oil (Nagle-Smith, 2024).

I first really paid attention to Ho wood when I heard aromatherapist Rehne Burge talk about it in her work with clients who had endured abuse. I find in my clinical work it is a soothing comforter that will cherish you: 'Ho wood helps you feel safer, taking the edge off angry, raw or heightened emotions. It is a wonderful antidote to what can feel like an increasingly violent and chaotic world' (Nagle-Smith, 2024, p.136).

Cautions

There are no known contraindications, but it should be noted that it can be confused with other chemotypes (e.g. ct. camphor). Tisserand and Young (2014) state that although it contains up to 1% of potentially carcinogenic constituents, on average it contains up to 80% of anticarcinogenic constituents, such as linalool and nerolidol.

Juniper berry (*Juniperus communis*)

Juniper comes from the family Cupressaceae and grows as a shrub or tree. The essential oil is steam distilled from Juniper berries. It is known for its anti-inflammatory, antimicrobial, antispasmodic and diuretic qualities, and is useful for rheumatic pain. Battaglia (2018) cites Holmes, who says it is useful for mental fogginess and self-confidence.

In the past, it was burnt as a way of cleansing from disease, and it has been thought to be spiritually protective.

Elizabeth Guthrie (2023) says she likes juniper for people who are struggling to trust their intuition and actions (which may happen to some people after trauma). She says, 'I generally find it helpful for people who are worrying so much it sends them into a freeze, or dorsal vagal response' (Guthrie, 2023, p.75).

In a YouTube vlog with Adam Barralet, author Elizabeth Ashley talks about her experience many years ago when she was in a domestic abuse situation. She mentions that Juniper helped ground her when she felt as if she wanted to disappear or dissociate (Barralet & Ashley, 2023).

Cautions

Many aromatherapy books state that Juniper should not be used by anyone with kidney problems and that it should be avoided in pregnancy. Tisserand and Young (2014) state it is possible that this is due to previous confusion between Junipers. That said, there are other clinically evidenced essential oils that can be used in pregnancy instead (Conrad, 2019).

Lavender (*Lavandula angustifolia*)

Lavender is probably the first essential oil that people think about when they consider aromatherapy. It is relatively low cost and is distilled from the plant's beautiful bluey purple flowers. It has a distinctive floral smell, which for some noses can be quite strong (in which case blending it works well). It is also the most researched essential oil, and has been shown to have analgesic, anti-allergic, anti-inflammatory, antinociceptive, tissue healing, antimicrobial and antioxidant and antispasmodic qualities (Rhind, 2020).

It is often used for first aid in terms of bites and stings, and the power of it was witnessed through a first aid response – a chemist called Gatefossé burnt his hand and plunged it into Lavender as the nearest liquid and was amazed at how quickly it healed. He coined the term aromatherapy. It can also act as emotional first aid and can be an aromatherapeutic 'rescue remedy' in times of shock. It was used in the past for panic and hysteria (Mojay, 1997). Mojay (1997) tells us that the almost closed-in flowers symbolize the level of self-protection and calm that the essential oil can induce. Various studies have shown it to reduce the stress hormone cortisol, reduce anxiety (without some of the side effects that anti-anxiety medication brings) and, in some instances, be sedative. Lavender, like some other essential oils, can modulate GABAergic transmission (gamma-aminobutyric acid (GABA) is the main inhibitory neurotransmitter in the central nervous system) (Rhind, 2020).

When my granny had her stroke (on her first birthday after my grandad's death), she was rushed to hospital. Unable to speak and move much, she was understandably frustrated, frightened and agitated. My mum would often place a single drop of Lavender on her nightgown. This would soothe and calm my granny during her difficult time, and if you have read my first book (Nagle-Smith, 2020) you will know that a huge lavender bush grew in her back garden next to the washing line. The smell was familiar to her and probably reminded her of the home she lived in for decades. My mum also uses Lavender essential oil a lot and, as such, I am sure this helped her too.

Cautions
There are no known hazards or contraindications according to Tisserand and Young (2014).

Lemon (*Citrus limonum*)
With a distinct and recognizable fresh, clear, light, zingy, slightly sweet, slightly sour aroma, Lemon is a very recognizable member of the Rutaceae family. It is very cheap and easy to source and became a panacea

in times of old for infection (Mojay, 1997). While it can be distilled or expressed, in aromatherapy we tend to use expressed essential oil.

Energetically it is cool and dry, associated with the earth element and often used for decongesting, cleansing and detoxing (Mojay, 1997). It is highly antiviral, and useful in sickrooms and for coughs and colds when people are run down and vulnerable, making them susceptible to becoming ill. *In vivo* and *in vitro* studies demonstrate it has antimicrobial, antitumoral, neuroprotective, anti-inflammatory, antioxidant and antinociceptive effects, and can relieve nausea and vomiting and enhance skin penetration. It is stress-relieving and can reduce anxiety and depression, but it can also be very useful as a study/learning aid, helping with memory (Rhind, 2020). As it is such a familiar smell to many, it can be helpful for bringing people into the present moment, and will sometimes make people's mouths water, putting them more in touch with their body.

Mojay (1997) tells us that it calms the busy mind, uplifts the intellect (Yi in Traditional Chinese Medicine), dissolves confusion, brings clarity and fosters trust and security, saying it can help open the heart and quell the worry of becoming overly emotionally involved.

Cautions
It is mildly phototoxic so skin shouldn't be exposed to sunlight or sunbeds for 12 hours after dermal application. Old and oxidized essential oils should be avoided. Do not use dermally at more than 2% (Tisserand & Young, 2014).

Neroli (*Citrus x aurantium*)
Neroli belongs to the Rutaceae family and is distilled from the flowers. It is incredibly expensive though its light floral aroma is very widely liked by everyone in my experience. Rhind (2020) provides the most beautiful description of it I have ever read. She says it has:

> a light, ethereal, floral top note with the faint impression of crushed green leaves, and a slightly bitter citrus note – maybe even lily-of-the-valley notes – all giving the initial impression of freshness and light – but in a short time, heady, more sensual 'orange blossom' notes will emerge. (Rhind, 2020, p.558)

Research with the essential oil suggests it is helpful for somatic anxiety and stress, and cardiovascular responses to stress via the autonomic nervous system. It also has pain-relieving and anti-inflammatory properties that can be useful for people experiencing long-term painful inflammatory conditions as a potential result of their trauma (Rhind, 2020). Rhind cites Weiss (1997), who noted that in traditional medicine, inhaling warm vapours was said to induce a trance-like state.

I refer to it as a hug in a bottle. I'm not sure if other people have called it this, or where this comes from, but it encompasses its personality beautifully. When you need comfort and support, when you are shocked and despairing, Neroli comes to the rescue.

I particularly like to use it when people have lacked a positive mother or mother figure in their lives and when they feel they need to be cared for. Bosson (2019) notes that both the essential oil and hydrolat calm shock and depression and work well for people in crisis, enabling calm communication. In the last chapter, we saw how beneficial Neroli hydrolat was for Nicole's clients when blended with Rose hydrolat. Baudoux (2020) describes it as being able to 'drive out dark thoughts', helping to support a deep, unbroken sleep and harmonizing and balancing the central nervous system. Guthrie (2023) says it imbues a sense of hope.

Cautions
There are no known cautions or contraindications (Tisserand & Young, 2014).

Orange (*Citrus sinensis*)
Orange (often known as Sweet orange) is from the family Rutaceae and the essential oil comes from the expressed rind. Orange is an incredibly familiar smell to many of us. It is normally loved, especially by children, and often brings back memories. In the UK, we would buy huge navel oranges specially for Christmas, or my mum would buy them in the summer holidays. When I peel an orange, I burst the rind (and thus the tiny ducts that hold the essential oil), releasing a wonderful aroma that still evokes happy memories of times gone by spent with family.

It may be useful for the respiratory system, constipation in particular and, with its antibacterial and anti-inflammatory nature, for the skin. Research shows it has an anxiolytic effect, so it is great for reducing anxiety. Rhind (2020) cites one study by Igarashi *et al.* (2014) that showed that women who inhaled either Orange or Rose (*Rosa damascena*) essential oil for 90 seconds demonstrated a noteworthy decrease in oxyhemoglobin concentration in the right prefrontal cortex, thus implying increased relaxed and comfortable feelings.

It is antispasmodic and carminative and from a Traditional Chinese Medicine perspective it unblocks stagnant Qi that can build up in the stomach, liver and intestines (Mojay, 1997). I like it with Roman chamomile (*Chamaemelum nobile/Anthemis nobilis*) or Curry leaf (*Murraya koenigii*), where there are emotional blockages mirrored by activity in the stomach. I find it useful for perfectionists and those who work and push themselves too hard, which can sometimes happen when people feel the need to keep busy so they don't stop and process trauma that has occurred for them.

I particularly like it blended with Cardamom (*Elettaria cardamomum*) for a feeling of warmth and being safely cocooned, especially if people feel cold and neglected. If they feel in need of a mothering oil (perhaps because they experienced a lack of love in the past or even now), I like to add Neroli (*Citrus x aurantium*). I also use it with Juniper (*Juniperus communis*) when someone needs calm confidence, motivation and the strength to carry on.

Cautions
There may be skin sensitization if old or oxidized essential oils are used. If it is included in products, an antioxidant should be used (Tisserand & Young, 2014).

Palo santo (*Bursera graveolens*)
Native to South America, Palo santo was used by the Incas. The essential oil comes from the distillation of the heartwood, and the tree comes from the family Burseraceae, like Frankincense (*Boswellia carteri*) and Myrrh (*Commiphora myrrha*). Denise Cusack told me she would use this essential oil with refugees from Mexico as it would smell familiar to them.

It is often thought that Palo santo is not sustainable. It is true that the tree has to be dead for several years before producing what is required for incense or the essential oil, and Peru currently has a ban on logging, but it is currently stated as being stable according to the IUCN (n.d.). In addition to this, there is another species, *Bulnesia sarmientoi*, which is also commonly known as Palo santo, and it may be that certain countries even have sub-species (Garzuglia, 2006). It is useful for joint pain, inflammation and muscle spasm and relaxation. I also use it with digestive issues such as irritable bowel syndrome that are made worse with stress and worry, and often seem to be present when someone has undergone trauma.

Warner (2018) recommends Palo santo for psychic protection, especially for people working in places where there might be lots of negative energy. She calls it 'spiritual disinfectant' and suggests healers wash their feet with it.

Cautions

Tisserand and Young (2014) state there may be issues with skin sensitivity if oxidation occurs. Due to the high limonene content, they recommend Palo santo be stored in an airtight container in the fridge. Any products blended using this essential oil would need to have an antioxidant added. According to them, maximum dermal use should be 3.4% because of the menthofuran and pulegone effects (both are hepatotoxic in large doses and the former has been shown to be lung toxic in rodents).

Roman chamomile (*Chamaemelum nobile/Anthemis nobilis*)

This is a perennial plant from the family Asteraceae, with a sweet fruity note. It reminds me of hay and overcooked sultanas, but many say it has an apple-like element in its aroma. In aromatherapy, we also use another Chamomile (*Chamomilla recutita/Matricia chamomilla*), commonly known as German chamomile, Blue or True chamomile. Both are relatively cheap and commercially easy to obtain. The latter shares many characteristics with Roman chamomile.

I prefer to use Roman chamomile for pain, spasm and where there are issues with the gut, and tend to use German chamomile more for skin issues, especially where there is heat energetically (in Traditional Chinese Medicine terms) underlying this.

Of Roman chamomile, Baudoux (2020) tells us that the plant was sacred to the pharaohs of Egypt and druids in Europe. It is powerfully analgesic, antispasmodic, anti-inflammatory, calming, soothing and sedative, and especially good for pain from spasm and neuralgia.

I find it very helpful when people feel physically tight, rigid and constricted (especially if they have been unable to sit still or have been pushing themselves physically or mentally in a frustrated or aggressive way). Roman chamomile helps you let go and surrender to slowing down. I particularly like it with Everlasting (*Helichrysum italicum*) and Clary sage (*Salvia sclarea*) for pain (especially migraines and headaches), and in helping people drift off to sleep, dispersing worries that are keeping them awake, and stopping the cycle of rumination. I wouldn't use it with Clary sage if I knew someone was using alcohol or antidepressants, as Clary sage can be very strong for some people, especially if they are quite sensitive, and it occasionally has an almost euphoric effect – I have witnessed a couple of people acting as if they are slightly drunk after using it. Baudoux (2020) indicates it for anger, irritability, agitation, excitement, psychological trauma and shock.

Holmes (2016) suggests it is a useful essential oil for anxiety, depression, panic attacks, PTSD and any condition that is made worse by stress. Mojay (1997) notes it is useful when tension resides in the solar plexus.

Battaglia (2018) cites Loughran and Bull (2001), who state it speaks to who we are. They connect it to expressing spiritual truth and the heart chakra. Kerkhof (2023) says it supports communication and is helpful for injuries to the soul, distress and grief.

Cautions
There are no known hazards or contraindications.

Rose (*Rosa damascena*)
Warner (2018) calls Rose the queen of oils. It is an incredibly expensive essential oil due to the number of petals required to produce just a tiny amount of essential oil. It belongs to the family Rosaceae. There are a few rose essential oils available but in aromatherapy we mostly use Rose otto, which is sometimes called Turkish rose (*Rosa damascena*) and Cabbage/Provence rose (*Rosa centifolia*). Absolutes are also available but are inferior.

Rose has an unmistakable sweet floral aroma. In the UK and USA, aromatherapists seem to report it is seen as less desirable by younger people, who often associate it with old people. In other cultures, and with different age groups, this may be different, as noted earlier by Denise and Nicole in their work. Warner (2018) notes that in different religions Rose and its scent has symbolized the sacredness of people's souls and/or that spiritual holiness was close by. Roses have been used to symbolize love and the heart for centuries.

Rhind (2020) notes that there is research to suggest it is analgesic, anxiolytic, antidepressant, hypertensive, decreases salivary cortisol, and supports the sympathetic nervous system. She cites Rakhshandah *et al.* (2004), who suggest its hypnotic effect is due to its affinity with the GABA system (Rhind, 2020).

Deby Atterby writes, 'Rose is the oil for the emotional heart. It is harmonizing, lifts the spirits and lightens the burden of sorrow' (Atterby, 2021, p.274).

Rose is often used by aromatherapists to soothe, open the heart and help manage traumas such as grief and any sort of loss or fear. She is a balm for wounds that you feel deep in your heart. Aromatherapists all seem to agree that Rose has a deeply feminine spirit.

Journeying with Galbanum (Ferula galbaniflua) *and Rose*
Writing this book has been extremely difficult at times. I would use a blend of 10% Rose diluted in 90% Jojoba oil on acupressure point C17. She was a gentle essential oil that journeyed with me, sitting hand in hand with me to help calm my soul as I read statistics about various abuses, explored personal experiences, researched, or feared that what I wrote would not do the subject justice. She reassured me and stayed with me until I felt confident enough to carry on, and she reminded me to stay present and not to get lost.

When I got really stuck and felt resistance, I used a drop of Galbanum on a tissue and he would give me the jolt to keep going forwards, even when I felt that I desperately wanted to retreat or couldn't write what needed to be written.

I could rarely work with Galbanum by himself, he was too overpowering. I would always have to reach for my Rose. Like a caring mother, Rose would then take the forcefulness from Galbanum and let me move more freely, gently encouraging me, just like a child being encouraged through the school gates on their first day.

As a synesthete, I see Rose as a deep magenta colour (like Jasmine (*Jasmine officinale var. grandiflorum*) and Ylang ylang (*Cananga odorata*)). Galbanum is a strong, bright emerald green, and the colour would rush forward first with the pink following behind at a slower pace and slowly submerging into the edges of the green. Seeing the essential oils in this way helped me understand and process their role.

Cautions
This may contain methyl eugenol, so maximum dermal use is 0.6% (Tisserand & Young, 2014).

Rosemary (*Salvia Rosmarinus*)

Please note that the Latin name for Rosemary has recently been changed from *Rosmarinus officinalis* to *Salvia Rosmarinus* (RHS, n.d.). Rosemary is steam distilled from the tops of the plant and belongs to the family Lamiaceae. There are several chemotypes, with *Salvia Rosmarinus ct. 1,8-cineole* being the most popular. The warm, dry herbaceous smell is familiar to many due to its use in cooking and herb gardens.

It has become known as the herb of remembrance, and has been used in weddings, funerals and sacred ceremonies. It was thought to be protective, warding off illness or evil spirits, and has become associated with improving the memory (Atterby, 2021).

It is useful for respiratory conditions, musculoskeletal pain and more, with its analgesic, antinociceptive, antispasmodic, anti-inflammatory, antihypertensive, expectorant, antibacterial and antidepressant properties (Rhind, 2020). Interestingly, it has been suggested that it may regulate the activities of the hypothalamic-pituitary-adrenal (HPA) axis and sympathetic nervous system (Villareal *et al.*, 2017, cited in Rhind, 2020). It comes into its own for focus and mental stimulation, and studies have shown it is useful in cognitive tasks such as remembering things (Rhind, 2020). This may be beneficial if memory is compromised after trauma and there is brain fog. Guthrie (2023) finds it is a favourite essential oil with some of her clients who are looking to assist their short-term memory. She recommends blending it with Bergamot (*Citrus bergamia/Citrus aurantium ssp. bergamia*) to create 'relaxed alertness'.

Emotionally, it is helpful for tension and loss of motivation (Rhind 2020), and can restore confidence and increase low self-esteem (Mojay, 1997). I find it brings a warmth and joy to the soul. As it sometimes reminds people of the Mediterranean, this may be meaningful if using it as an anchor.

Cautions

Avoid if you are pregnant. Do not apply to (or near to) the face of infants or children (Tisserand & Young, 2014). Avoid during fevers and use at no more than 2% (Mojay, 1997). People who have epilepsy should avoid Rosemary. It is also contraindicated for people who are hyperactive, hypervigilant or restless. Prolonged use is best avoided if someone is vulnerable, frail or taking multiple medications. Avoid dermally when someone has high blood pressure (Kerkhof, 2023).

Vetiver (*Chrysopogon zizanioides*, formerly known as *Vetiveria zizanioides*)

Vetiver is a grassy plant that is native to India, and from the family Poaceae. If you have never seen a picture of Vetiver, I urge you to take a look. The essential oil comes from its dramatically long roots. It is even used in certain parts of the world to help erosion as its fine net of roots is useful in binding soil (Rhind, 2020). These roots and the rhizome are steam distilled to produce the essential oil we use. It comes from various parts of the world, including Réunion (often reputed to be the best), China, Java, India, America, Madagascar and Haiti.

It has a deep, earthy aroma, that most people like or dislike. I love it and in my mind's eye, I associate Vetiver with colours of dark earth.

Rhind (2020) notes it may be useful for the integumentary system, especially for things like dermatitis, acne, wound healing and the muscular skeletal system (e.g. for inflammation, arthritis, rheumatism and pain). Some animal experiments showed refreshing or stimulating effects too (Rhind, 2020).

Vetiver is sometimes used in study blends; however, I have always found it really helpful for sleep, especially where there is difficult and stubborn insomnia. It is deeply grounding and can be very comforting where there is distress, especially if paired with an oil that comforts and soothes such as Rose (*Rosa damascena*) or Neroli (*Citrus x aurantium*). I also like it with Ylang ylang (*Cananga odorata*) to impart confidence in one's body and ability to manage things. I find it can be very powerful and often only 1 drop in a blend is required.

Battaglia (2021) tells us that it has a cooling energy, and many associate it with the base or root chakra. It can be applied to the solar plexus for protection.

Cautions

Vetiver from Java, China, Brazil and Mexico contains isoeugenol and therefore should not be used at more than 1.5% dermally according to the International Fragrance Association (Tisserand & Young, 2014).

Yarrow (*Achillea millefolium*)

Yarrow is from the family Asteraceae. The plant is thought to be named after Achilles who is said to have used yarrow to tend to the wounds inflicted by battle, and it has an ethnobotanical use of stemming bleeding. As there are many chemotypes around the world, Rhind (2020) points out that it is hard to postulate the benefits, but these should include being pain relieving, helping digestive cramps and spasms, providing immune support and easing respiratory inflammation and congestion.

For me, Yarrow comes into its own when it is used for psychological wounds or unspoken hurt and change, when there are disenfranchised emotions, or it feels as if there are fragmented parts of the self, and we are left asking who am I now? What remains of me? It can be very useful during transitions, times of change or when people are questioning their role in life, wondering how they got to where they are at or feeling as if they don't know who they are anymore. I have also found it useful for clients who experience such feelings due to hormonal changes in perimenopause.

Battaglia (2018) recommends using Yarrow with Cypress (*Cupressus sempervirens*), Fragonia (*Taxandria fragrans*), Neroli (*Citrus x aurantium*) or Everlasting (*Helichrysum italicum*) when there is change, and states it is associated with the throat chakra (Battaglia, 2021). Warner (2018) recommends it for psychic protection.

Cautions
There is a risk of drug interaction (e.g. with drugs metabolized by CYP2D6), so do not use dermally if someone is taking medication (see note 1 earlier in the chapter).

Ylang ylang (*Cananga odorata var. genuina*)
Ylang Ylang is a tropical tree that produces exquisite yellow flowers which are fractional steam distilled to produce essential oil. Each 'fraction' has a slightly different composition and smell. It has a heady, tropical, quite intense aroma (which I find similar to the intensity of Jasmine (*Jasmine officinale var. grandiflorum*)). Adding it to other oils that can modulate its aroma can be useful, such as woody oils or Nagarmotha (*Cyperus scariosus*) or Violet leaf (*Viola odorata*).

While it may be useful for mild acne and musculoskeletal tension, it really comes into its own for nervous tension, stress, anxiety, frustration and confidence in the body's ability to cope. When people have panic attacks or are triggered, it often leads them to want to avoid situations and it can erode confidence. In such instances, I have found Ylang ylang to be very helpful. It may be useful blended with Lavender (*Lavandula angustifolia*) for panic attacks.

Annoyingly, it is often referred to as being useful for 'frigidity' – a term I hate and think should never be used because it is often used in a bullying, misogynistic, traumatizing way that leads to sexual grief. The essential oil does have the benefit of uniting the mind and body, which can be helpful if someone feels unconfident in intimacy or struggles with their relationship with the more intimate parts of their body.

Cautions
There is a moderate risk of skin sensitization, so do not use on hypersensitive, diseased or damaged skin. Maximum dermal use is 0.8%. It should not be used with children under two years old (Tisserand & Young, 2014).

INFUSED/MACERATED OILS

These are normally diluted and added into balms, butters or body lotions. They are usually diluted by being added to a carrier oil. I normally do a maximum of 5ml infused oil to 25ml of carrier oil.

Arnica infused oil (*Arnica montana*)
Arnica comes from the family Asteraceae and is a perennial herb. It is analgesic, anti-inflammatory, and is useful for mental fatigue, restlessness, agitation, insomnia and night sweats. Interestingly, it is also indicated for hair loss due to trauma or anxiety.

Cautions
Care should be taken if someone already has sensitivity to the Asteraceae family. Do not use for long periods of time as it can cause irritation, and do not use on areas of broken skin.

Calendula/Marigold (*Calendula officinalis*)
Marigolds have long-held traditions in many cultures and several religions. In South America, the flowers are used on the day of the dead, when ancestors who have passed are remembered, and the flowers were sacred to the Aztecs. Traditionally, they have also been used for divination, psychic dreams, protection and prophecy work. The flower is generally thought of as bringing warmth and positivity and is sometimes called the herb of the sun. Please note, it is very different to Tagetes.

Warner (2018) states it can provide protection (including protection from our or others' negative emotions), balance and support when there is grief, fear, heartache and emotional trauma. She says it is useful for providing insight. While she is talking about the essential oil, I feel many of the subtle, energetic benefits of the plant transfer when the blooms are macerated in oil (which is how we get Calendula infused oil).

More recently, I have used a CO_2 total extract. This can be more challenging to work with as it is a thick consistency (rather like marmite). I find the best thing to do is pop some in a cup, then put the cup into a larger bowl of very warm water and stir, then add in the carrier oil and continue to stir. The warmth and stirring should distribute it nicely. I find 2–5% in sunflower oil is often sufficient if using it for its emotional and spiritual aspects. I find it stains less and I can buy it in very small amounts, which are easier to keep than a larger bottle of infused oil.

It is useful for skin care, especially eczema and scars and wounds that struggle to heal well. Aromatherapist Madeleine Kerkhof (2018) tells us that the CO_2 extract is superior for wound healing, nourishing, skin regenerating, soothing and enhancing skin hydration; it is also fungicidal and anti-inflammatory.

It can be very helpful in blends, along with other carrier oils when someone's trauma has made their skin condition worse.

Cautions
It can stain clothing and massage couch linen, although in low dilution with the CO_2 extract I have not noticed any staining (but do not rely on my experience, just in case!).

St John's wort (*Hypericum perforatum*) infused oil
St John's wort has bright yellow flowers and the oil is a deep red colour. Like many other infused oils, it is anti-inflammatory, wound healing and analgesic. It is also useful where there are spasms and pain due to neuromuscular diseases (Kerkhof, 2023), which are often traumatic for those experiencing them. St John's wort is also helpful for nerve issues and sciatica, especially ones that come from stressful situations. I have sometimes found that sciatica can be a painful side effect of regularly being sat at someone's bedside (often due to sitting at strange angles, on hard chairs in hospitals for long periods of time). It is indicated for nervous tension, restlessness, insomnia, debility, anxiety and depression.

Cautions

As it is phototoxic, avoid exposure to sunlight or sunbeds for 12 hours after it is diluted and used on the skin. Unlike the herbal preparations which are taken internally, it does not interfere with other medication when applied topically and diluted on the skin.

Finding what works for you/your clients

In your aromatic journey, you will always find your favourites. I struggled to narrow this down as there are so many more aromatic friends that I could have included, such as Sweet marjoram (*Origanum majorana*; though I prefer a CO_2 to the essential oil). It is so calming and helpful when there are pent-up emotions, overthinking or spasms. Peppermint (*Mentha x piperita*) is also beneficial for clients who need to focus mentally or who need to digest new ways of being so they can move forwards. I have written about Iary (*Psiadia altissima*), Katafray (*Cedrelopsis grevei*) and Kunzea (*Kunzea ambigua*) in my previous two books and in journals but I find them very supportive. Violet leaf (*Viola odorata*) absolute is useful when the trauma is related to extreme grief or watching a loved one's demise, and Elemi (*Canarium luzonicum*) is helpful for letting go. Melissa (*Melissa officinalis*) is also useful when depression is entrenched. There are many more, including comforting Benzoin (*Styrax tonkinensis*) and Cardamom (*Elettaria cardamomum*), Myrrh (*Commiphora myrrha*) and Sandalwood (*Santalum austocaledonicum*) to still the mind, and Cypress (*Cupressus sempervirens*) to help with all manner of transitions.

Most importantly, it is about finding what is right for the individual. As aromatherapist Rehne Burge says, 'Trauma is not a 'one shoe fits all' topic...neither are the remedies.'

Reflection points

- If you are new to aromatherapy, has this chapter given you some ideas of essential oils you would like to try?
- If you are trained as an aromatherapist, many of these oils will be very familiar to you but perhaps with trauma in mind, are you now thinking about them with a slightly different lens? And is there a new aromatic ally you would like to investigate?

CHAPTER 9

Looking after your client and yourself

Choose mindful and compassionate action.

Guthrie, 2022, p.313

By engaging with an aromatherapist, clients are proactively trying to reach (or maintain) a state of homeostasis. This is something we applaud and wish to help them do. Our intention should always be for the higher good and not to do harm, which is why I like the above quote from Elizabeth Guthrie so much.

However, to support our clients, it is important that we too maintain our own equilibrium. Many complementary therapists (myself included if I am honest) often struggle to do this but it is essential. I often remind my clients of the phrase we hear so often on airplanes, 'Fit your own oxygen mask before fitting anyone else's.' This chapter will address additional support for both parties.

Supporting our clients
Relaxation, grounding and being present
As aromatherapists, we can be part of our client's resource and be someone who supports them in feeling safe. We can help them feel centred, grounded and more body aware.

Haines (2016) uses the mnemonic OMG (orient, move and ground) as a way of exploring how people who've experienced trauma can manage when they feel activated. I find this very helpful as a concept because it encompasses what many complementary therapists try to do in their work with individuals. So, let us break down what he means.

Orientation, Haines reminds us, is about being in the here and now.

Being with the people and space around you. One commonly used exercise for this is the 5,4,3,2,1 exercise which encompasses all the senses. It involves, for example, naming five things that can be seen (e.g. furniture, signs, pictures, plants, my watch), four things that can be felt (e.g. feet in shoes, clothes on skin, jewellery, bottom on the chair), three things that can be heard (e.g. a bird tweeting, a car driving past, a plane in the sky), two things you can smell (e.g. perfume, body lotion), one thing you can taste (e.g. coffee, a sip of water, toothpaste from when you brushed your teeth, a sweet, chewing gum). One of my clients was taught this by her psychotherapist and she tells me she finds this especially useful when feelings become overwhelming.

Movement, Haines tells us, is about being aware of your body and expanding in your space. He suggests that a tiny movement, such as wriggling toes or moving the hands together or visualizing running, can be helpful. When we work with our clients, we help them become more aware of their body and what feels comfortable, different, safe, unusual and changed.

When someone feels tense and finds it hard to let go, I find that asking them to bring their shoulders up to their ears, clench them tight and then breathe out and let go can be useful. Sometimes, I now ask clients if they want to shake things out a bit before they get onto the massage couch.

People often hold themselves stiffly, so if you can encourage them to have more ability to change how their body feels through movement they can find this very empowering. If you are interested in harnessing the power of the body and inhabiting the body more fully, I recommend reading *Humanal* by Betsy Polatin (2020).

Grounding, Haines says, can be achieved by self-talk and awareness of simple things like the sensations of our feet on the ground, or being able to feel where our body meets the chair. When my aromatherapy massage clients lie down on the massage couch, I sometimes (depending on the scenario) suggest they take some slow comforting breaths and feel themselves lying comfortably on the couch. I may expand this and ask them to extend their awareness to where the couch makes contact with their body, or where the sheets lie on their skin.

There are many useful grounding exercises that can be done, and as we have already seen, smelling an aroma can be anchoring and grounding. I find essential oils that come from trees (bark or resin) especially useful for this, but it is a very individual matter. The smell of a commonly loved herb such as rosemary, a strong pungent smell such as peppermint, or a familiar enjoyable fruit (such as orange) can often help people feel more present, more rooted and grounded.

In the Mind video (2016) I mentioned earlier in the book, one of the participants said that when she starts to dissociate, her friends will notice and get her an ice lolly as she finds the change in temperature helps bring her back. She also mentioned how the smell of Lavender (*Lavandula angustifolia*) or a strong-smelling hand cream help her.

During the COVID-19 lockdowns I continued to work with some clients remotely via Zoom. I was able to demonstrate and guide them on self-massage and I used relaxation and grounding techniques to keep them in the present and in touch with their bodies. During this time, people were often stressed, worried and, in some instances, traumatized.

One very simple grounding exercise can be to ask someone to consider their body as they sit in a chair. It might go something like this:

- If you feel comfortable to do so, close your eyes. If you prefer to leave your eyes open, you can maintain a soft gaze. You may wish to let your arms fall by your sides or place your hands on your lap, whatever works best for you.
- Take a few comfortable breaths and just be in this moment.
- Feel your feet placed firmly on the floor, making contact with the ground, grounding you.
- Feel where your body meets the chair, where your back and thighs make contact.
- Note any sensations that you feel on your skin such as the fabric of your clothes or material that the chair is made from. Maybe you feel a flow of air from a window or heater, or the warmth of the sun through a window or from a lamp.
- Take a few moments and note what you observe. Just be here.

Depending on the situation, I might then progress this further and take their attention to different parts of their body from their head, right down to the toes (this is often known as a body scan). Asking them to consider how each part feels, I start with the scalp and end with the heels, soles of the feet and toes. Towards the end of this I say something like:

- Feel how grounded you are in this moment. Enjoy this realization. Now slowly give your fingers and toes a wriggle, and in a moment, we will gently open our eyes.

I am then silent for a moment.

- Allow that beautiful feeling of being grounded to stay with you, and when you are ready, slowly open your eyes.

There are many grounding techniques that can be done either in person or remotely. If you work remotely, you can even send an essential oil or blend to your client beforehand.

So many of us live in our heads, it is incredibly helpful to be reminded to consider how other parts of our body may feel. Importantly, it is also helpful for people to consider sending some energy, love, kindness, recognition or positive touch to areas of the body that feel as if they need more support. They can do this by placing their hands on that part of their body if that feels comfortable for them, or they can envisage sending love or a positive colour or breath to that area. Doing this while working with an essential oil that promotes self-love and compassion such as Rose (*Rosa damascena*) or Neroli (*Citrus x aurantium*) can be very powerful.

It is important to remember that a small percentage of people are unable to visualize (they can't see things in their mind's eye, or day-dream, for example), so if someone tells you they can't do anything that includes visualization, consider other tools they may find useful.

I have also found that some people really struggle to relax. In fact, sometimes being asked to relax can evoke a negative or physical reaction (such as stiffening). In my work, I avoid the word 'relax' with people who have medical trauma, as they are often told to do this just before a horrible medical procedure. We all know that if we are told to 'just relax', it can be hard to do so. Sometimes we change our language. We might suggest that they let their arms go floppy or we may encourage someone to tighten and clench everything and then breathe out and 'let go'.

I noticed that the UK charity Rape Crisis (2023b), has a quite extensive list of grounding techniques on its website and I recommend looking at this for more ideas.

Aromatherapy and massage

As an aromatherapist who works using massage, I find there are ther-apeutic benefits to massage alone. This can then be amplified and extended by the introduction of aromatherapy. For example, if I feel a client is struggling to regulate, I find rhythmic rocking motions while the client lies face down can be useful. Some body workers do this with a hand, others use a forearm, others use their leg. It provides movement and rhythm into the body and can sometimes (though not always) help when someone has been holding themselves tightly in a defensive mode.

Slow, longer, sweeping movements using the forearm can feel very reassuring when we are trying to encourage a sense of slowing down because the body is in a hypervigilant state.

At the beginning of a session, I often ask people to take a few slow deep breaths. I ask them to be aware of their body making contact with the massage couch, feeling the drapes on their skin, the temperature of the room and so on. This can be useful for orientating themselves in their body. Also asking if they are aware of any places in their body that feel soft or safe can help if they feel nervous, or are struggling to relax.

When clients are lying on their backs, face up on a massage couch they are normally lying in Savasana, a well-known restorative yoga pose. For years, I have been encouraging my clients to spend a few minutes a day if possible adopting this pose at home (many prefer a bolster or rolled towel underneath the knees, especially if they suffer with back-ache). It has a dual purpose – first and most importantly, it allows the body to rest, relax and restore; second, many of my clients spend a lot of time sitting at a computer or on a laptop. Gravity and the nature of the posture means that their shoulders naturally go back towards the mat/floor, and their neck is lengthened.

Breathing

Many people don't breathe well. Betsy Polatin (2020) reminds us that if a child feels like crying but tries not to, they will hold their breath, so we should remember this when working with clients who are distressed or have cried a lot. Trauma often seems to impact breathing.

I've had instances where a client (in both past and current careers) has said they are about to tell me something they haven't told anyone else. Before doing so there is often a big inhale/gulp of air and then a holding of the breath, before whatever is said comes tumbling out. After crying or sobbing, it can take them quite some time to regulate their breathing, but we can help people do this through co-regulation. If they hear and see us breathing slowly and deeply, they can often fall into this pattern with us. It is why it is so important in first aid (including mental health first aid) and trauma work to stay calm and steady, so you can help the other person.

Poor breathing can become habitual and brings about its own problems such as a longer-term form of hyperventilation syndrome (sometimes called a breathing pattern disorder), where the person breathes faster and/or deeper. As too much carbon dioxide gets exhaled, this changes adrenaline levels and increases heart and breathing rate (University Hospital Southampton NHS Foundation Trust, 2023). People with this often complain of tension in their neck and shoulders, and if you work on the chest, they will discover that they have sensations of tightness here and that many of the chest muscles feel a bit sore. Please note though, that in some cases, symptoms can mimic heart problems, so if in doubt, a person should always seek medical attention.

We can ask our clients to explore how they are breathing (whether they are with us in person, or we are seeing them virtually). They can do this by placing one hand on their chest and one hand on their belly and assessing which hand moves the most. I prefer people to do this lying down though it can be done seated.

Thinking outside the box and adapting how we work

It is important to allow ourselves to think outside the box and reflect on the tools we can give clients, while maintaining boundaries and staying within our professional remit.

Sometimes we can change simple things we do, like adapting our consultation forms, taking greater note of someone's posture when they come for an appointment, starting with a simple grounding technique or asking them to observe their breathing (or doing this ourselves). Sadly, these things are not always taught in all aromatherapy courses.

I recently wondered how powerful it would be for someone to be able to mark on a diagram of the human body areas where they felt discomfort. They could even colour this in. Over the weeks, they could repeat this exercise each time so we could see what had changed. It is something that never occurred to me before, but it can be a helpful visualization. It also says a lot when it is hard to verbalize. Other measures can also be used, including MYMOP® (Measure Yourself Medical Outcomes Profile).[1]

Jonathan Benavides found a lovely way of thinking outside the box and continuing to support his clients during the global trauma of COVID-19. He used an A3 photograph of a forest alongside a 'forest' blend of essential oils (12 drops of it were given to the client on an inhaler aroma stick). The blend was designed to relax, and help the client's respiratory system, and release any tension. He encouraged the client to sit for ten minutes using his forest essential oil blend and

---

1   www.meaningfulmeasures.co.uk

the forest photo whenever they needed to. It is a great example of finding a way to adapt so something aromatically meaningful can still occur (Benavides, 2021).

Blending aromatherapy with other modalities

You can include aroma in the other modalities you offer, if you feel you are able to stay within the remit of your role, it is agreed by your professional body and your insurance, and you do no harm. For example, I know many people who are trained as aromatherapists but are also trained yoga or pilates teachers, reiki or reflexology practitioners. We saw this in the Chapter 7 with Elaine's dual role with reiki, chakras and aromatherapy.

For example, I like to incorporate a few acupressure points, such as CV17, when there is anxiety, sorrow, sadness, grief or a feeling of despair. To find this on yourself, you can put the fingertips of one hand on your breastbone (your little finger should be on the bottom of the breastbone), or GV24.5 when there is emotional unease. This point is effectively where we consider the 'third eye' to be. Reed Gach (1990) notes that this point is indicated for chronic fatigue, depression and irritability.

I like to lay a finger on the GV24.5 point and then travel my fingers backwards in a line over the top of the head. This encompasses other useful points such as GV19, GV20 and GV21 as well. If this is something you feel drawn to there are many teachers worldwide who provide courses, but there are also some good books for the lay person, including *Acupressure: How to Cure Common Ailments the Natural Way* by Michael Reed Gach (1990).

Really engaging with smelling the essential oil

As an aromatherapist, I constantly come up against the idea that aromatherapy is simply nice smells. To move beyond this preconception we can consider the usefulness of aroma as an anchor, and also deeply involve our client in their ability to connect with their sense of smell.

One of the ways we can do this is by asking people to smell a single essential oil or blend and sit with it. In a busy world, especially when the mind is frantic, this can be challenging, so you may be met with a little resistance occasionally. For example, we can ask someone to inhale an essential oil (e.g. on a smelling strip), and then ask them to continue to inhale several times.

When they smell it, ask them what immediately comes to mind. It may be words, a visual image, a memory. It may smell familiar or new.

If they focus on the aroma, where does that aroma go in their body? When they smell it, do they notice any differences in their mind or body anywhere? For example, someone smelling Peppermint (*Mentha x piperita*) or Eucalyptus (*Eucalyptus globulus*) will often say they feel as if they can breathe more deeply and as if their nose expands. Does the smell go anywhere in particular in their body? For example, with Peppermint and Eucalyptus, people often say the smell goes into their head and their lungs and it expands outwards. With essential oils like Angelica root (*Angelica archangelica*), Cedarwood (*Cedrus atlantica*) and Nagarmotha (*Cyperus scariosus*), people are more likely to feel that it takes them downwards.

If they are a visual person, they might imagine a colour or sound that the aroma might have. Really getting them to engage in the aroma they are smelling and focusing on this sense can be a powerful way of helping someone feel present. They can continue this at home and even write about it if they wish. By purposefully engaging our sense of smell, we naturally encourage ourselves to be in our bodies.

Simple things such as going on a walk and being aware of the different smells we can smell as we walk can also help us stay present and be more aware of our body.

In 2023, I went on a course run by Elizabeth Ashley and Deby Atterby. During the course we did a walking meditation in a figure of eight, walking the 'infinity' symbol. This was intriguing to me because I had never considered not being still while doing a meditation. It occurred to me on this day that adding this rhythmic movement was surprisingly soothing. This reminded me of how trauma expert van der Kolk (2014) notes that there are many different activities that enable us to have agency, from athletics to drama and expressive arts. It is finding what works for the individual, and movement may be part of that.

The figure of eight also reminded me of how Peter Levine (1997) discusses trauma and healing vortexes. He states that when we revisit and re-enact trauma, we can get pulled into a trauma vortex. However, healing can come through a counter vortex being produced, and we can move back and forth between the two states in a figure of eight pattern until the energies disperse. If you are a visual person, you may appreciate the subtleties and similarities of this.

The role of synaesthesia
Incidentally, a small proportion of the population are synaesthetic (meaning they involuntarily combine two or more senses). If someone

tells you a smell tastes, sounds, looks or feels a certain way, encouraging them to embrace this is very powerful. This is part of their true self.

Those with synaesthesia often learn early in their cognitive journey that most of the world doesn't sense things quite like they do, and this ability may be ridiculed or seen as weird. As aromatherapists, we should be supporting them in enjoying this part of themselves. It can be very interesting for them to explore their reactions to an aroma, and to some extent most people who can smell can extend the way in which they combine and think about their senses to appreciate aroma on a slightly different level.

Interestingly, Ward (2020) theorizes that synaesthesia may make someone more vulnerable to PTSD. He cites earlier research (Chin & Ward, 2018) that demonstrates that synaesthetes are more likely to remember events through an 'own eyes' perspective, which is also known as a first-person perspective. In non-synesthetes, he points out, this is more linked to emotionally significant events. Furthermore, the synaesthesia may make rewriting traumatic memories more challenging. Much more research is necessary to test this theory, but it is something to bear in mind (Ward, 2020).

Encouraging clients to check in with their body

When we see our clients for appointments, we commonly ask things like 'How are you?' and 'How has your week been?' and 'How are you feeling?' We note their posture and observe their body language as well as the words they use and their tone of voice. I sometimes wonder how much clients check in with themselves in between appointments. We can encourage them to do this by asking questions about which parts of the body feel safe, calm, at ease or comfortable.

We can also ask them if they notice any areas of the body where there is a tension or tightness. They may verbalize this or show you using hands or by pointing. This helps them become more aware of their body and informs your work. How much do our clients connect with themselves in this way outside their appointments? Encouraging them to try this exercise at home daily or journalling on this may be useful for some people.

After I read Betsy Polatin's (2020) book, I noticed I was suddenly much more aware of areas of my body that felt as if they had been squashed or constricted. I had only started to consider this, because I had been made to consistently consider how my body flexed, moved and how I held myself. In fact, when I heard her talk in 2023, I remember her saying that just the effort of standing for some people is simply a lot. I was momentarily surprised, but then I thought about it. Ordinary, everyday things can still be difficult for some people, especially when they have experienced trauma.

Other practices clients can try at home
Many cultures, religions and traditions adopt practices that involve sounds or words, singing or humming. These can be quite regulating, rhythmic and soothing. Levine (The Master Series on Trauma Conference, 2023), for example, suggests making the sound *oooooo* (so it sounds like a really long 'you' but without the y). Menakem (2021) suggests repeating the word *Om* (so it stretches into three syllables). Perhaps your clients have other tools they use to help them soothe and regulate? Menakem also explores how humming, some singing (especially lullabies or anything with repetition) and even rocking gently can be a way for some people to successfully soothe. Some practices may be carried out with a willing friend or family member, for example, humming together, taking a walk with someone and then falling into step together, taking it in turns to massage each other's hands (Menakem, 2021).

For aromatherapists, holistic and complementary therapists
Maintaining professional boundaries
We may work with clients in our remit as aromatherapists, but we should remember to stay within the parameters of our role and not to give advice on things we are not trained for. This means that we do not give medical advice or advise on things like nutrition if we are not qualified and insured to do so. Working with trauma is no different. We must always remember that our remit is aromatherapy. It is our responsibility to 'do no harm'. That means we don't become someone's counsellor or tell them that we can heal their trauma.

Knowing when to refer on and being honest with yourself
Referring a client either to another aromatherapist or another professional can be tricky. If done well, it can provide the client with the required support, done badly it can leave them feeling alone, let down and even abandoned. It should always be done professionally and carefully.

A good starting point is communicating sensitively what you think might be useful and explaining why. Allowing your client choice is important too. Many services will accept a self-referral. If a referral from a doctor or someone else is required, you can ask your client if they would like you to write to the person who can make the referral (but make it clear to the person you are referring to that your client has given you written permission to do this). If you are unsure, always take advice from your professional body or insurance company on this.

Your client should have a copy of any such correspondence, and you should add it to their client record/notes. In the UK, they legally have the right to request a copy of these (Information Commissioner's Office, 2024). It is important to make very detailed client notes that demonstrate what discussion was had with your client, the agreed outcome and the actions taken.

Many people who have experienced trauma have been in situations where they have had their choice and control taken away from them, so it is important to continue to allow them to have this choice. If they choose not to take up your suggestion of a referral, accept that this is their right. Do not berate them or keep asking them to seek help from another professional – it will probably only continue a cycle of shame.

Breaking confidentiality

This can feel very difficult for some aromatherapists because they feel that their client trusts them, but it is important to know and understand the law in respect to this, and the code of your professional body. This may differ from country to country so understanding what legalities surround this in the country you work in is necessary.

You can involve your client in this process (as discussed earlier in the book), explaining why you need to break confidentiality (e.g. that you are concerned for their safety), and considering how best to do this together. Again, you need to keep detailed client records as regards the conversation about breaking confidentiality, agreed action, outcomes, any follow up required.

Having a support system/debriefing

As mentioned in Chapter 6, having a trusted mentor/aromatherapy buddy with whom you can hold a debrief after a difficult situation with a client is extremely helpful. It needs to be a relationship where there is trust and confidentiality and you need to be careful not to share identifying information. You may even belong to a small group of professionals where you can do this.

Cleansing your workspace

Cleansing the room/space you work in can be useful, especially when the room feels heavy with emotion. In such instances, I like to air the room well, use music or an essential oil. You may have other rituals you do to help.

Looking after yourself

There are many ways we can look after ourselves and maintain good levels of self-care. An obvious one that many of us forget to do when we are in a rush or busy is to simply check in with ourselves before and after seeing a client. Asking yourself, 'How am I feeling right now?' can provide great insight.

I find I prefer to take showers rather than baths after a day of seeing clients. As the water rushes off me, I imagine any residual negative energy being washed away. Water has a long history of being spiritually cleansing.

During a conference on trauma in 2023, one of the participants who was a psychotherapist asked Stephen Porges what he suggested people do to avoid secondary trauma when working with someone who is traumatized. He suggested they spend time with an animal or person who is not part of that world, co-regulating with them to get social connection and support. Taking a walk, playing a sport, gardening and other hobbies are simple ways people can focus on one task to cleanse the mind and body.

As we have seen, recognizing our own wounds and working on our own personal growth and healing journeys are also important. This shouldn't be viewed as a 'one off' but a continuous journey. We always have more to learn.

Being with people who raise your energy and support you in a loving way can be nurturing. As we spend a lot of time looking after other people it is important not only to look after ourselves, but also to allow ourselves to be looked after so we can recalibrate. If there aren't people (or enough people) in your life who do this, consider what action you could take to help change that.

US clinical aromatherapist Jade Shutes reminded me one day that connection with the earth and growing things can be a powerful tool in helping where there is a trauma history. Being outdoors and among plants can be very grounding.

As she mentioned this, I pondered on the fact that I had powerfully felt the need to take on an allotment as I started my research on this book. I knew I needed somewhere to go and 'escape', a place where I could just be. The plot would continue to grow with or without me. There was no pressure to be a certain way, no need to talk or behave in a particular way. If I worked it, I felt the benefits emotionally. All I needed to do was be there. It didn't ask anything of me. Having somewhere where you can 'just be' and having a connection with the earth can be very useful.

Essential oils, hydrolats and CO_2 extracts can be powerful agents connecting us to both plant life and the world at large, establishing our bonds to the life cycle of the plant and mother nature's bounty. Like our sense of smell, they are a precious gift for our clients and ourselves.

Reflection points

- Do you have a good support network and a safe space to self-reflect on your work with others?
- Do you make time for your own self-care?

CHAPTER 10

Final thoughts

We are on the verge of becoming a trauma-conscious society.

van der Kolk, 2014, p.417

Writing this book, I have realized the extent of the intimate relationship between memory, our sense of smell, trauma, physiology and the brain in general. I had been aware to some extent, but hadn't really understood the complexities, nuances and wider implications.

The consequences of what we now know about trauma, our bodies (including our sense of smell) and our brains need to shape what we do next to move forwards as a trauma-informed society. For those of us who are aromatherapists, it also needs to shape our work.

Now that we realize the olfactory process is affected by trauma (especially developmental trauma), we can support people in this. Aromatherapists (and others) can ask clients questions about their ability to smell, and we can support those struggling by offering smell training.

Aromatherapists and others need to have a greater voice in communicating the importance of our sense of smell within society. As trauma ripples through society, we need to help people understand *why* and *how* olfaction is such a useful sense. As we have seen, essential oils and aromas are used in exposure therapy in the world of traumatology, as well as creatively and compassionately by aromatherapists in many settings around the globe, including refugee camps, substance abuse centres, children's homes, hospitals, hospices, special education needs schools, disaster zones, in private practice, with veterans, and more. Essential oils are a helpful, low cost, accessible tool and they can be used alongside other treatment such as talking therapies or EMDR.

However, I do believe that the world of traumatology and polyvagal theory would be greater enhanced by really embracing where smell sits in the conversation. As our understanding of the body and theories around trauma and physiology expand we may see more connections being made. There is much more to learn. For example, I am intrigued by the thought that when we smell, we may 'feel' the aroma in our nose and throat. Should we be considering that odour perhaps can be 'felt' on some level as well as smelt? There is still so much we do not understand about our olfactory system and, as such, odours may have a greater impact on our mind and body than we currently realize.

I remain hopeful that we can enhance our understanding of trauma and how it affects our lives, appreciating its very impact on us all both individually and collectively, and that we can move forwards with great compassion and kindness. Our aromatic allies, such as essential oils, will be there to help us.

I thank you, the reader, for your interest in aroma, aromatherapy and trauma, and I hope you will take this knowledge forwards in a way that will benefit others.

Support organizations

Support for those affected by loss of smell and taste
Absent. Support with olfaction – www.abscent.org

Anosmia Awareness. Support for those affected by the loss of the sense of smell – www.anosmiaawareness.org

Association Anosmie. American non-profit organization to spread awareness for those without the sense of smell – www.anosmie.org

Fifthsense. A charity dedicated to smell and taste disorders, covering France, Belgium, Spain, Luxembourg, Quebec and Morrocco – www.fifthsense.org.uk

Smell and Taste Association of North America (STANA). A voice for people with smell and taste disorders through education and public awareness – https://thestana.org

Support with trauma
Assist Trauma Care. Specialist not-for-profit organization based in the UK – https://assisttraumacare.org.uk

Birth Trauma Association. UK charity dedicated to supporting women and families who have experienced traumatic birth – www.birthtraumaassociation.org

Combat Stress. A UK charity for the mental health of veterans – https://combatstress.org.uk

Cruse. UK charity providing bereavement support – www.cruse.org.uk

Mind. For people who have, or are living with someone who has, a mental health issue. UK based – www.mind.org.uk

NAPAC (The National Association for People Abused in Childhood). UK charity supporting adult survivors of abuse – https://napac.org.uk

PTSDUK. UK-based charity raising awareness of PTSD – www.ptsduk. org

Rape Crisis. Feminist charity in England and Wales working to end sexual violence and abuse – https://rapecrisis.org.uk

UK Trauma Council. Supporting professionals, communities and policy makers through resources and guidance in responding to traumatic events that impact on children and young people – https:// uktraumacouncil.org/research-practice/research-round-up

Bibliography

Action for Children (2023) *60% rise in parents and carers seeking help for school refusal from action for children's parent talk service*. Available at www.actionforchildren.org.uk/media-centre/seeking-help-for-school-refusal (Accessed 29/01/24).

Andrews, K., Lloyd, C.S., Densmore, M., Kearney, B.E. *et al.* (2023) 'I am afraid you will see the stain on my soul': Direct gaze neural processing in individuals with PTSD after moral injury recall. *Social Cognitive and Affective Neuroscience*, 18(1), 1–11.

Arshamian, A., Gerkin, R.C., Kruspe, N., Lundström, J.N., Mainland, J.J. & Majid, A. (2022) The perception of odour pleasantness is shared across cultures. *Current Biology*, 32, 2061–2066.

Ashley, E. (2016) *Helichrysum – For the Wound that Will Not Heal*. The Secret Healer.

Atterby, D. (2021) *Australian Essential Oil Profiles*. Elanora, Australia: AAT Publishing.

Bailey, R., Dugard, J., Smith, S.F. & Porges, S.W. (2023) Appeasement: Replacing Stockholm syndrome as a definition of survival strategy. *European Journal of Psychotraumatology*, 14(1), 2161038.

Barralet, A. & Ashley, E. (2023) *Juniper Berry*. Available at www.youtube.com/watch?v=kxbMXfRkLSY (Accessed 03/02/24).

Barwich, A.S. (2020) *Smellosophy*. Cambridge, MA: Harvard University Press.

Battaglia, S. (2018) *The Complete Guide to Aromatherapy. Vol I – Foundations and Materia Medica*. Third edition. Brisbane, Australia: Black Pepper Creative.

Battaglia, S. (2021) *The Complete Guide to Aromatherapy. Vol III – Psyche and Subtle*. Third edition. Brisbane, Australia: Black Pepper Creative.

Baudoux, D. (2020) *Contemporary French Aromatherapy*. London: Singing Dragon.

Benavides, J. (2021) What is going to happen to me next? Aromatherapy in pandemic times. *International Journal of Clinical Aromatherapy*, 15(1 & 2), 3–7.

Benavides, J. (2023, 20–21 May) *Aromatic support for improving body image post-mastectomy*. Essence of Clinical Aromatherapy Conference, Edinburgh.

Bhat, Z.A., Kumar, D. & Shah, M.Y. (2011) Angelica *archangelica* Linn. is an angel on earth for the treatment of diseases. *International Journal of Nutrition, Pharmacology, Neurological Diseases*, 1(1), 36–50.

Birkmayer, F. (2022) Essential oils for the wounded healer: PTSD, post traumatic resilience and the wounded healer's journey. *International Journal of Professional Holistic Aromatherapy*, 11(3), 37–41.

Blades, J. (2021) *Making It: How Love, Kindness and Community Helped Me Repair my Life*. Basingstoke: Bluebird.

Blakey, S.M., Wagner, H.R., Naylor, J., Lane, I. *et al.* (2018) Chronic pain, TBI and the PTSD in military veterans: A link to suicidal ideation and violent impulses? *The Journal of Pain*, 19(7), 797–806.

Boesveldt, S. & Parma, V. (2021) The importance of the olfactory system in human well-being, through nutrition and social behaviour. *Cell and Tissue Research*, 383(1), 559–567.

Bosson, L. (2019) *Hydrosol Therapy*. London: Singing Dragon.

Britannica, The editors of Encyclopaedia (2023) *Hurricane Katrina*. Available at www.britannica.com/event/Hurricane-Katrina (Accessed 14/12/23).

Britannica, The editors of Encyclopaedia (2023) *Japan earthquake and tsunami of 2011*. Available at www.britannica.com/event/Japan-earthquake-and-tsunami-of-2011/Aftermath-of-the-disaster (Accessed 14/12/23).

Buck, L. & Axel, R. (1991) A novel multigene family may encode odorant receptors: A molecular basis for odor recognition. *Cell*, 65(1), 175–187.

Charlton, E. (2023) Peer support. *In Essence*, 22(1), 62.

Cobb, M. (2020) *Smell*. Oxford: Oxford University Press.

Conrad, P. (2019) *Women's Health Aromatherapy*. London: Singing Dragon.

Cortese, B.M., Leslie, K. & Uhde, T.W. (2015) Differential odour sensitivity in PTSD: Implications for treatment and future research. *Journal of Affective Disorders*, 1(179), 23–30.

Croy, I., Symmank, A., Schellong, J., Hummel, C., Gerber, J., Joraschky, P. & Hummel, T. (2014) Olfaction as a marker for depression. *Journal of Affective Disorders*, 160, 80–86.

Cruse (n.d.) *Growing around grief*. Available at https://www.cruse.org.uk/understanding-grief/effects-of-grief/growing-around-grief (Accessed 31/01/24).

Cruse (2023) *Traumatic grief*. Available at www.cruse.org.uk/understanding-grief/grief-experiences/traumatic-loss/traumatic-grief (Accessed 14/12/23).

Daniel, D.R. & Zolnikov, T.R. (2023) The use of bergamot essential oil for PTSD symptomology: A qualitative study. *American Journal of Qualitative Research*, 7(4), 1–32.

Davis, P. (2005) *Aromatherapy – An A–Z*. London: Vermilion.

Day, J & P. (n.d.) Fragonia® Information Sheet. The Paperbark Co. Available at https://paperbarkoils.com.au (Accessed 23/10/20).

Debiec, J. & Sullivan, R.M. (2014) Intergenerational transmission of emotional trauma through amygdala-dependent mother-to-infant transfer of specific fear. *Proceedings of the National Academy of Sciences of the USA*, 111(33), 12222–12227.

Dias, B.G. & Ressler, K.J. (2014) Parental olfactory experience influences behaviour and neural structure in subsequent generations. *Natural Neuroscience*, 17(1), 89–96.

Docter-Loeb, H. (2023) *The study of smell loss still struggles for support*. Available at https://undark.org/2023/09/27/smell-loss-research (Accessed 04/12/23).

Eastholm, D. (2018) Effects of an essential oil blend on the symptoms of post-traumatic stress disorder. *International Journal of Professional Holistic Aromatherapy*, 6(4), 33–36.

Eliyan, Y., Wroblewski, K.E., McClintock, M.K. & Pinto, J.M. (2021) Olfactory dysfunction predicts the development of depression in older US adults. *Chemical Senses*, 1(46).

Elliot, D.E., Bjelajac, P., Fallot, R.D., Markoff, L.S. & Glover Reed, B. (2005) Trauma informed or trauma denied: principles and implementation of trauma informed services for women. *Journal of Community Psychology*, 33(4), 461–477.

Ellis, C. & Knight, K.E. (2022) Advancing a model of secondary trauma: Consequences for victim service providers. *Journal of Interpersonal Violence*, 36(7–8), 3557–3583.

Emerald, M. (2016) Potential use of essential oils in prevention and management of PTSD. *International Journal of Professional Holistic Aromatherapy*, 4(4), 13–21.

Essentially Australia (2023) *Australian Rosewood*. Available at https://essentiallyaustralia.com.au/product/australian-rosewood-essential-oil (Accessed 03/02/24).

Fallout, R.D. & Harris, M. (2008) Trauma-informed approaches to systems of care. *Trauma Psychology Newsletter* (American Psychological Association), 3(1), 6–7.

Farruggia, M.C., Pellegrino, R. & Scheinost, D. (2022) Functional connectivity of the chemosenses: A review. *Frontiers in Systems Neuroscience*, 16, 865929.

Felitti, V.J., Anda, R.F., Nordenberg, D., Williamson, D.F. *et al.* (1998) Relationship of childhood abuse and household dysfunction to many of the leading causes of death in adults. The Adverse Childhood Experiences (ACE) study. *American Journal of Preventative Medicine*, 14(4), 245–258.

Fifth sense (2023) *How smell works*. Available at www.fifthsense.org.uk/how-smell-works (Accessed 09/11/23).

Fischer-Rizzi, S. (1990) *Complete Aromatherapy Handbook*. New York, NY: Sterling Publishing.

Fisher, J. (2023) *Module 2: treating the scars of abandonment*. Mastering the treatment of trauma, online seminar. National Institute for the Clinical Application of Behavioral Medicine 11/10/23.

Galia, F. (2023) The Smell Gym. Available at www.smellgym.com (Accessed 18/01/24).

Garzuglia, M. (2006) *Threatened, endangered and vulnerable tree species: A comparison between FRA and IUCN Red list*. Available at https://openknowledge.fao.org/items/2d8a81ce-d439-4628-bdeb-e80155489e4a (Accessed 25/05/24).

Golla, M. (2017) Essential oils: Warming the soul in crisis situations. Pflege Professionell. Available at https://pflege-professionell.at/de-aetherische-oele-seelenwaermer-in-krisensituationen (Accessed 17/12/23).

Grossman, S., Cooper, Z., Buxton, H., Hendrickson, S. *et al.* (2021) Trauma-informed care: recognizing and resisting re-traumatization in health care. *Trauma Surg Acute Care*, 6(1), e000815.

Guthrie, E. (2022) *The Trauma Informed Herbalist*. Self-published.

Guthrie, E. (2023) *Essential Oils for Trauma*. Self-published.

Haines, S. (2016) *Trauma Is Really Strange*. London: Singing Dragon.

Hakim, M., Battle, A.R., Belmer, A., Bartlett, S.E., Johnson, L.R. & Chehrehasa, F. (2019) Pavlovian olfactory fear conditioning: Its neural circuitry and importance for understanding clinical fear based disorders. *Frontiers in Molecular Neuroscience*, 12, 221.

Hassan, R. & Nettleton, M. (2023) *Trauma informed coach certificated course*. Module 1 The Centre for Healing. Available at www.thecentreforhealing.com (Accessed 17/08/24).

Heaton-Shrestha, C. (2022) Perspectives on integrating aromatherapy with psychotherapeutic counselling and psychotherapy – a preliminary enquiry. *International Journal of Professional Holistic Aromatherapy*, 11(3), 5–17. https://www.ijpha.com/back-issuesbooks.

Hedrich, W.D., Hassan, H.E. & Wang, H. (2016) Insights into CYP2B6-mediated drug-drug interactions. *Acta Pharmaceutica Sinica B*, 6(5), 413–425.

Herman, J.L. (2023) *Truth and Repair*. London: Basic Books.

Herz, R.S. (2021) Olfactory virtual reality: A new frontier in the treatment and prevention of posttraumatic stress disorder, *Brain Science*, 11(8), 1070.

Herz, R.S. & Bajec, M.R. (2022) Your money or your sense of smell? A comparative analysis of the sensory and psychological value of olfaction. *Brain Science*, 12(3), 299.

Hinton, D.E., Pich, V., Chhean, D., Pollack, M.H. & Barlow, D.H. (2004) Olfactory-triggered panic attacks among Cambodian refugees attending a psychiatric unit. *General Hospital Psychiatry*, 26(5), 390–397.

Holmes. P. (2016) *Aromatica Volume 1*. London: Singing Dragon.

Holmes. P. (2019) *Aromatica Volume 2*. London: Singing Dragon.

Holy Bible (2011) *Holy Bible*. New International version. London: Hodder & Stoughton.

Hummel, T. & Podlesek, D. (2021) Clinical assessment of olfactory function. *Chemical Senses*, 46, bjab053.

Illig, K.R. & Wilson, D.A. (2009) 'Olfactory Cortex: Comparative Anatomy.' In L.R. Squire (ed.), *Encyclopedia of Neuroscience* (pp.101–106). Oxford: Academic Press.

IUCN Red List (n.d.) *Bursera graveolens*. Available at www.iucnredlist.org/search?query=palo%20santo&searchType=species (Accessed 25/05/24).

IUCN Red List (2020) *Rosewood*. Available at www.iucnredlist.org/species/61795859/617959 06#geographic-range (Accessed 23/12/23).

IUCN Red List (2023) *Atlas Cedar*. Available at www.iucnredlist.org/species/42303/ 2970716#taxonomy (Accessed 21/12/23).

Jeong, H.J., Leighton Durham, E., Moore, T.M., Dupont, R.M. *et al.* (2021) The association between latent trauma and brain structure in children. *Translational Psychiatry*, 11(1), 240.

Karolinska Institutet (2022) *People around the world like the same kinds of smells*. Karolinska Institute. Available at https://news.ki.se/people-around-the-world-like-the-same-kinds-of-smell (Accessed 26/10/23).

Katrinli, S., Oliveira, N.C.S., Felger, J.C., Michopoulos, V. & Smith, A.K. (2022) The role of the immune system in posttraumatic stress disorder. *Translational Psychiatry*, 12(313). https://doi.org/10.1038/s41398-022-02094-7.

Kerkhof, M. (2018) *CO² Extracts in Aromatherapy*. The Netherlands: Kicozo.

Kerkhof, M. (2023) *Clinical Aromacare*. The Netherlands: Kicozo.

Koyama, S. & Heinbockel T. (2020) The effects of essential oils and terpenes in relation to their routes of intake and application. *International Journal of Molecular Science*, 21(5), 1558.

Langley-Brady, D.L., Shutes, J., Vinson, J.J. & Zadinsky, J.K. (2023) Aromatherapy through the lens of trauma-informed care: Stress-reduction practices for healthcare professionals. *Journal of Interprofessional Education & Practice*, 30, 100602.

Levine, P. (1997) *Waking the Tiger*. Berkeley, CA: North Atlantic Books.

Levine, P. (2018) 'Polyvagal Theory and Trauma.' In S. Porges & D. Dana (ed.) *Clinical Applications of the Polyvagal Theory*. New York, NY: W.W. Norton and Company.

Lewis, D. & Ossola, A. (2023) How smell is helping treat the toughest cases of trauma. *Wall Street Journal*. Available at www.wsj.com/podcasts/wsj-the-future-of-everything/how-smell-is-helping-treat-the-toughest-cases-of-trauma/08c7b400-0f9f-45c5-af34-e69a51a4c35f (Accessed 24/11/23).

Lewis, S.J., Arseneault, L., Caspi, A., Fisher, H.L. *et al.* (2019) The epidemiology of trauma and post-traumatic stress disorder in a representative cohort of young people in England and Wales. *The Lancet Psychiatry*, 6(3), 247–256.

Lewis-O'Connor, A., Warren, A., Lee, J.V., Levy-Carrick, N. *et al.* (2019) The state of the science on trauma inquiry. *Women's Health*, 15, 1–17.

Lizarrange-Valderrama, L.R. (2021) Effects of essential oils on central nervous system: Focus on mental health. *Phytotherapy Research*, 35, 657–679.

Lizarraga-Valderrama, L.R. (2023) Pharmacological effects of essential oils. *In Essence* (IFPA Journal), 22(1), 36–40.

Lykkegaard Ravn, S. & Andersen, T.E. (2020) Exploring the relationship between posttraumatic stress and chronic pain. *Psychiatric Times*, 37(11), 19–21.

Mackereth, P. & Carter, A. (2022, 20–22 May) Anosmia, Aroma and Acupressure. Botanica 2022 conference (online).

Mackereth, P., Carter, A. & Maycock, P. (2023) Aromatic calm techniques (ACTs) for needle anxiety and phobia. *International Journal of Professional Holistic Aromatherapy*, 11(4), Spring, 15–20. https://www.ijpha.com/back-issuesbooks.

Maté, G. (2019) *When the Body Says No*. London: Vermilion.

Maté, G. & Maté, D. (2023) *The Myth of Normal*. London: Vermilion.

Menakem, R. (2021) *My Grandmother's Hands*. London: Penguin.

Mind (2016) *Dissociation*. Available at www.youtube.com/watch?v=UvhtDZ7G6jI (Accessed 12/12/23).

Mojay, G. (1997) *Aromatherapy for Healing the Spirit*. Rochester, VT: Healing Arts Press.

Mortensen, J. (2023) Vagus nerve stimulation with essential oils: A brief review. *International Journal of Professional Holistic Aromatherapy*, 11(4), 37–39.

Munyan, B.G., Neer, S.M. & Beidel, F.J. (2016) Olfactory stimuli increase presence in virtual environments. *PLoS ONE*, 11(6), e0157568.

Murphy, F., Nasa, A., Cullinane, D., Raajakesary, K. *et al.* (2022) Childhood trauma, the HPA axis and psychiatric illnesses: A targeted literature synthesis. *Frontiers in Psychiatry*, 13, 748372.

Nagle-Smith, H. (2020) *Working with Unusual Oils; An Aromatic Journey with Lesser Known Essential Oils*. Vol 1. Self-published.

Nagle-Smith, H. (2024) *Working with Unusual Essential Oils*. London: Singing Dragon.

National Institute for Health and Care Excellence (NICE) (2018) *Post-traumatic stress disorder*. Available at www.nice.org.uk/guidance/ng116/chapter/Recommendations (Accessed 29/01/24).

National Institute for Health and Care Excellence (NICE) (2023a) *When should I suspect post-traumatic stress disorder (PTSD)?* Available at https://cks.nice.org.uk/topics/post-traumatic-stress-disorder/diagnosis/diagnosis (Accessed 10/12/23).

National Institute for Health and Care Excellence (NICE) (2023b) *Scenario: Management of adults and children with post-traumatic stress disorder*. Available at https://cks.nice.org.uk/topics/post-traumatic-stress-disorder/management/management/#psychological-therapies-drug-treatment (Accessed 10/12/23).

National Institute for the Clinical Application of Behavioural Medicine (NICABM) (n.d.) *How to help your clients understand their window of tolerance*. Available at www.nicabm.com/trauma-how-to-help-your-clients-understand-their-window-of-tolerance (Accessed 31/01/24).

Native Extracts (2023) *Rainforest blue oil*. Available at www.nativeextracts.com/products/rainforest-blue-essential-oil (Accessed 03/02/24).

Nayeri, D. (2019) *The Ungrateful Refugee*. Edinburgh: Canongate Books.

Newcomb, M., Burton, J., Edwards, N. & Hazelwood, Z. (2015) How Jung's concept of the wounded healer can guide learning and teaching in social work and human services. *Advances in Social Work and Welfare Education*, 17(2), 55.

NHS Scotland (2021). *Trauma informed practice: Toolkit*. Available at www.gov.scot/publications/trauma-informed-practice-toolkit-scotland/documents (Accessed 29/01/24).

NSPCC (2023) *Child protection plan statistics: England 2019–2023*. Available at https://learning.nspcc.org.uk/research-resources/child-protection-plan-register-statistics (Accessed 25/01/24).

Pieniak, M., Oleszkiewicz, A., Avaro, V., Calegari, F. & Hummel, T. (2022) Olfactory training – thirteen years of research reviewed. *Neuroscience and Biobehavioural Reviews*, 141, 104853.

Polatin, B. (2020) *Humanual: A Manual for Being Human*. San Diego, CA: Waterside Productions.

Porges, S.W. (2009) The polyvagal theory: New insights into adaptive reactions of the autonomic nervous system. *Cleveland Clinical Journal of Medicine*, 76(2) S86–S90.

Porges, S.W. (2022) Polyvagal theory: A science of safety. *Frontiers in Integrative Neuroscience*, 16, 871227.

Porges, S.W. & Dana, D. (ed.) (2018) *Clinical Applications of the Polyvagal Theory*. New York, NY: W.W. Norton and Company.

Porges, S.W. & Porges, S. (2023) *Our Polyvagal World*. New York, NY: W.W. Norton and Company.

Porter, J., Craven, B., Khan, R.M., Chang, S.J. *et al.* (2007) Mechanisms of scent tracking in humans. *Nature Neuroscience*, 10(1), 27–29.

Price, A. (2021) The power of aromatherapy massage to nurture resilience: A personal perspective. *International Journal of Clinical Aromatherapy*, 15(1&2), 3–10.

PTSDUK (2023a) *Symptoms of post-traumatic stress disorder and C-PTSD*. Available at www.ptsduk.org/what-is-ptsd/symptoms-of-ptsd (Accessed 25/09/23).

PTSDUK (2023b) *The science and biology of PTSD*. Available at www.ptsduk.org/what-is-ptsd/the-science-and-biology-of-ptsd (Accessed 25/01/23).

PTSDUK (2023c) *Complex PTSD (C-PTSD)*. Available at www.ptsduk.org/what-is-ptsd/complex-ptsd (Accessed 08/02/24).

PTSDUK (2023d) *Prolonged exposure therapy and PTSD*. Available at www.ptsduk.org/prolonged-exposure-therapy/ (Accessed 11/12/23).

PTSDUK (2023e) *Causes of post-traumatic stress disorder*. Available at www.ptsduk.org/what-is-ptsd/causes-of-ptsd (Accessed 25/01/23).

Purchon, N. & Cantele, L. (2014) *The Complete Aromatherapy and Essential Oils Handbook for Everyday Wellness*. Toronto: Robert Rose.

Raab, D. (2022) Are you a wounded healer? *Psychology Today*. Available at www.psychologytoday.com/gb/blog/the-empowerment-diary/202201/are-you-wounded-healer (Accessed 20/11/23).

Rabellino, D., Frewen, P.A., McKinnon, M.C. & Lanius, R.A. (2020) Peripersonal space and bodily self-consciousness: Implications for psychological trauma-related disorders. *Frontiers in Neuroscience*, 14, 586605.

Ranjbar, N., Erb, M., Mohammad, O. & Moreno, F.A. (2020) Trauma-informed care and cultural humility in the mental health care of people from minoritized communities. *Focus*, 18(1), 8–15.

Rape Crisis (2023a) *Rape and sexual assault statistics: Sources*. Available at https://rcew.fra1. cdn.digitaloceanspaces.com/media/documents/Rape_and_sexual_assault_statistics_ sources_February_2024_xM27tE0.pdf (Accessed 15/02/24).

Rape Crisis (2023b) *Grounding techniques*. Available at https://rapecrisis.org.uk/get-help/ tools-for-victims-and-survivors/grounding (Accessed 02/01/23).

Reed Gach, M. (1990) *Acupressure: How to Cure Common Ailments the Natural Way*. London: Piatkus.

Rhind, J.P. (2016) *Aromatherapeutic Blending*. London: Singing Dragon.

Rhind, J.P. (2020) *Essential Oils*. London: Singing Dragon.

RHS (n.d.) Rosemary becomes a sage. Available at www.rhs.org.uk/plants/articles/misc/ rosemary-becomes-a-sage (Accessed 04/06/2).

Rothschild, B. (2000) *The Body Remembers*. New York, NY: W.W. Norton and Company.

Schaal, B., Saxton, T.K., Loos, H., Soussignan, R. & Durand, K. (2020) Olfaction scaffolds the developing human from neonate to adolescent and beyond. *Philosophical Transactions Royal Society*, 375 (1800). https://doi.org/10.1098/rstb.2019.0261.

Schlinzig, T. (2021) Odour as a medium of cohesion and belonging. *Open Edition Journals. Sociology and Anthropology*, 52(1), 47s69.

Skipper, C. (2019) *The breath of Angelica*. Available at https://cathysattars.com/ the-breath-of-angelica/?v=79cba1185463 (Accessed 21/12/23).

Skipper, C. (2020a) *Ancestral healing transforms our current traumas*. Available at https:// aromagnosis.com/ancestral-healing-transforms-our-current-traumas (Accessed 03/12/23).

Skipper, C. (2020b) *Tools for healing trauma*. Available at https://aromagnosis.com/tools-for-healing-trauma (Accessed 03/12/23).

Skipper, C. (2022) *Angelica*. Available at www.youtube.com/watch?v=_EkcuhWWXmQ (Accessed 26/05/22).

Smith Hayduk, K. (2022) *Researchers reveal how trauma changes the brain*. Available at www. urmc.rochester.edu/news/publications/neuroscience/researchers-reveal-how-trauma-changes-the-brain (Accessed 13/11/23).

South East Fermanagh Foundation (2012) *Exploring the Effectiveness of Complementary Therapies on Trauma Related Illnesses*. Available at https://seff.org.uk/wp-content/ uploads/2020/11/THERAPIES-REPORT-2012-28th-JUNE.pdf (Accessed 17/08/24).

Stojanovic, M.P., Fonda, J., Brawn Fortier, C., Higgins, D.M. *et al.* (2016) Influence of mild traumatic brain injury (TBI) and posttraumatic stress disorder (PTSD) on pain intensity levels in OEF/OIF/OND veterans. *Pain Medicine*, 17(11), 2017–2025.

Tedeschi, R.G. & Calhoun, L. (2004) Posttraumatic growth: A new perspective on psycho-traumatology. *Psychiatric Times*, 21(4). Available at www.psychiatrictimes.com/view/ posttraumatic-growth-new-perspective-psychotraumatology (Accessed 18/12/23).

Teicher, M.H. & Samson, J.A. (2016) Annual research review: Enduring neurobiological effects of childhood abuse and neglect. *Journal of Child Psychology and Psychiatry*, 57(3), 241–266.

Tesarz, J., Baumeister, D., Andersen, T.E. & Bjarke Vaegter, H. (2020) Pain perception and processing in individuals with posttraumatic stress disorder: A systematic review with meta-analysis. *Pain Reports*, 5(5), e849.

The Master Series on Trauma Conference (2023, 31 August–3 September) https:// themasterseries.com/oxford-university-event, Oxford.

Tisserand, H. (2018) *Grapefruit Oil and Medication*. Tisserand Institute. Available at https:// tisserandinstitute.org/learn-more/grapefruit-oil-and-medication (Accessed 22/12/23).

Tisserand, R. (2017) Did you know that Copaiba oil makes your skin happy? Available at https://tisserandinstitute.org/learn-more/copaiba-oil (Accessed 08/05/24).

Tisserand, R. & Young, R. (2014) *Essential Oil Safety*. Edinburgh: Churchill Livingstone.

Totaro, P. & Wainright, R. (2022) *On the Scent*. London: Elliot and Thompson.

UK Government (2022) *Working definition of trauma informed practice*. Available at www. gov.uk/government/publications/working-definition-of-trauma-informed-practice/ working-definition-of-trauma-informed-practice (Accessed 13/11/23).

UK Trauma Council (2023a) *Trauma*. Available at https://uktraumacouncil.org/trauma/ trauma (Accessed 08/02/24).

UK Trauma Council (2023b) *Post-traumatic stress disorder (PTSD) and complex PTSD*. Available at https://uktraumacouncil.org/trauma/ptsd-and-complex-ptsd?cn-reloaded=1 (Accessed 13/11/23).

University Hospital Southampton NHS Foundation Trust (2023) *Breathing pattern disorders* Version 3. University Hospital Southampton NHS Foundation Trust.

van der Kolk, B. (2014) *The Body Keeps the Score*. New York, NY: Penguin.

Véscovi, C. (2022) Post-trauma healing with essential oils. *International Journal of Professional Holistic Aromatherapy*, 11(3), Winter, 43–48.

Waibel, J., Patel, H., Sidhu, R. & Lupatini, R. (2021) Prospective, randomized, double blind, placebo-controlled study on efficacy of Copaiba oil in silicone based gel to reduce scar formation. *Dermatology Therapy*, 11, 2195–2205.

Ward, A. (2023) *How smell – the most underrated sense – was overpowered by our other senses*. Available at https://lithub.com/how-smell-the-most-underrated-sense-was-overpowered-by-our-other-senses (Accessed 04/12/23).

Ward, J. (2020) Is synaesthesia a predisposing factor to post-traumatic stress disorder? *Frontiers in Bioscience–Scholar*, 13(1), 14–16.

Warner, F. (2018) *Sacred Oils*. London: Hay House.

Watson, C. (2018) *The Language of Kindness*. London: Vintage.

Weiss, T., Soroka, T., Gorodisky, L., Shushan, S., Snitz, K. *et al.* (2020) Human olfaction without apparent olfactory bulbs. *Neuron*, 105(1), 35–45.

Woods, L. & Farr, A. (2019) *Interview with Lisa Woods on behalf of BreakForth at CASS Art*, 24 April 2019. Available at www.andyfarr.com/twistedrose and https://youtu.be/26sbPSb48Gw (Accessed 22/01/24).

Youssef, N.A., Lockwood, L., Su S., Hao, G. & Rutten, B.P.F. (2018) The effects of trauma, with or without PTSD, on the transgenerational DNA methylation alterations in human offsprings. *Brain Sciences*, 8(5), 83.

Zhu, X., Suarez-Jimenez, B., Lazarov, A., Such, S. *et al.* (2022) Sequential fear generalization and network connectivity in trauma exposed humans with and without psychopathology. *Communications Biology*, 5, 1275.

Zilcha-Mano, S., Zhu, X., Lazarov, A., Suarez-Jimenez, B., Helpman, L. *et al.* (2022) Structural brain features signalling trauma, PTSD or resilience? A systematic exploration. *Depression and Anxiety*, 39(10–11), 695–705.

Zoll, L. & Davila, L. (2023) *Disenfranchised trauma: The impact on indirect victims*. Available at www.socialworker.com (Accessed 30/11/23).